QuickFACTS™

Basal and Squamous Cell SKIN CANCER

What You Need to Know—NOW

QuickFACTS™

From the Experts at the American Cancer Society

Basal and Squamous Cell SKIN CANCER

What You Need to Know—NOW

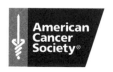

Published by the American Cancer Society/Health Promotions
250 Williams Street NW, Atlanta, Georgia 30303 USA

Copyright ©2012 American Cancer Society

For permission to reprint any materials from this publication,
contact the publisher at **permissionrequest@cancer.org**.

Printed in the United States of America
Cover designed by Jill Dible, Atlanta, GA
Composition by Graphic Composition, Inc.

5 4 3 2 1   12 13 14 15 16

Library of Congress Cataloging-in-Publication Data

Basal and squamous cell skin cancer : what you need to
    know—now / from the experts at the American Cancer
    Society.
        p. cm.—(Quick facts)
    Includes bibliographical references and index.
    ISBN 978-1-60443-039-4 (pbk. : alk. paper)
    ISBN 1-60443-039-7 (pbk. : alk. paper)
    1. Basal cell carcinoma—Popular works. 2. Squamous cell
carcinoma—Popular works. I. American Cancer Society.
RC280.S5B364 2012
616.99'477—dc22

                                              2011009547

Quantity discounts on bulk purchases of this book are avail-
able. Book excerpts can also be created to fit specific needs.
For information, please contact the American Cancer Society,
Health Promotions Publishing, 250 Williams Street NW,
Atlanta, GA 30303-1002, or send an e-mail to **trade.sales
@cancer.org**.

A Note to the Reader

This information represents the views of the doctors and nurses serving on the American Cancer Society's Cancer Information Database Editorial Board. These views are based on their interpretation of studies published in medical journals, as well as their own professional experience.

The treatment information in this book is not official policy of the Society and is not intended as medical advice to replace the expertise and judgment of your cancer care team. It is intended to help you and your family make informed decisions, together with your doctor.

Your doctor may have reasons for suggesting a treatment plan different from these general treatment options. Don't hesitate to ask him or her questions about your treatment options.

For more information, contact your American Cancer Society at **800-227-2345** or **cancer.org**.

TABLE OF CONTENTS

Your Skin Cancer

What Is Cancer?.............................1

What Are Basal and Squamous Cell
Skin Cancers? 3

Normal Skin 3

Types of Skin Cancer.......................5

Basal Cell Carcinoma........................6

Squamous Cell Carcinoma 7

Less Common Types of Skin Cancer 8

Precancerous and Preinvasive Skin Conditions 10

Benign Skin Tumors..........................12

What Are the Key Statistics About Basal and
Squamous Cell Skin Cancers? 12

Risk Factors and Causes

What Are the Risk Factors for Basal and Squamous
Cell Skin Cancers?............................15

Exposure to Ultraviolet Radiation 16

Fair Skin 17

Older Age 18

Male Gender 18

Exposure to Certain Chemicals.................18

Radiation Exposure 18

Previous Skin Cancer........................18

Long-term or Severe Skin Inflammation or Injury ...18

Psoriasis Treatment 19

Xeroderma Pigmentosum 19

Basal Cell Nevus Syndrome...................19

Reduced Immunity 19

Human Papilloma Virus Infection 20

Smoking 20

**Do We Know What Causes Basal and Squamous
Cell Skin Cancers?. 20**

Prevention and Detection

**Can Basal and Squamous Cell Skin Cancers
Be Prevented? 23**

Limit Exposure to Ultraviolet Radiation 23

Avoid Tanning Beds and Sunlamps 28

Protect Children from the Sun. 28

Sun Exposure and Vitamin D 28

Avoid Harmful Chemicals 29

Learn More About Skin Cancer Prevention 29

**Can Basal and Squamous Cell Skin Cancers
Be Found Early?. 30**

Diagnosis and Staging

**How Are Basal and Squamous Cell Skin
Cancers Diagnosed? 33**

Signs and Symptoms of Basal and Squamous
Cell Skin Cancers 33

Medical History and Physical Examination 35

Skin Biopsy 36

Examining the Biopsy Samples 37

Lymph Node Biopsy 37

**How Are Basal and Squamous Cell Skin
Cancers Staged? 38**

The American Joint Committee on Cancer
(AJCC) TNM System. 39

Stage Grouping 41

Treatment

How Are Basal and Squamous Cell Skin Cancers Treated? 43

Surgery 43

Other Forms of Local Therapy 46

Radiation Therapy 48

Systemic Chemotherapy 50

Clinical Trials. 52

Complementary and Alternative Treatments 59

Treatment of Basal Cell Carcinoma 63

Treatment of Squamous Cell Carcinoma 64

Treatment of Actinic Keratosis. 66

Treatment of Bowen Disease 67

Treatment of Merkel Cell Carcinoma. 67

Your Medical Team 68

More Treatment Information 69

Questions to Ask

What Should You Ask Your Doctor About Your Skin Cancer? 71

After Treatment

What Happens After Treatment for Basal and Squamous Cell Skin Cancers? 73

Follow-up Care 73

Seeing a New Doctor. 75

Lifestyle Changes to Consider During and After Treatment 75

Make Healthier Choices. .76

Latest Research

What Is New in Research and Treatment of Basal and Squamous Cell Skin Cancers? **77**

Basic Skin Cancer Research 77

Public Education 77

Preventing Genital Skin Cancers 78

Chemoprevention 78

Treatment. 79

Resources

Additional Resources **81**

More Information from Your American Cancer Society. 81

National Organizations and Web Sites. 82

References 82

Glossary   **85**

Index   **103**

Your Skin Cancer

What Is Cancer?

The body is made up of hundreds of millions of living cells. Normal body cells grow, divide, and die in an orderly fashion. During the early years of a person's life, normal cells divide faster to allow the person to grow. After the person becomes an adult, most cells divide only to replace worn-out or dying cells or to repair injuries.

Cancer* begins when **cells** in a part of the body start to grow out of control. There are many kinds of cancer, but they all start because of out-of-control growth of abnormal cells.

Cancer cell growth is different from normal cell growth. Instead of dying, cancer cells continue to grow and form new, abnormal cells. Cancer cells can also invade other **tissues**, something that normal cells cannot do. Growing out of control and invading other tissues are what makes a cell a cancer cell.

*Terms in **bold type** are further explained in the glossary, beginning on page 85.

Cells become cancer cells because of damage to **DNA**. DNA is in every cell and directs all its actions. In a normal cell, when DNA is damaged, the cell either repairs the damage or the cell dies. In cancer cells, the damaged DNA is not repaired, but the cell does not die like it should. Instead, this cell goes on making new cells that the body does not need. These new cells will all have the same damaged DNA as the first cell.

People can inherit damaged DNA, but most DNA damage is caused by mistakes that happen while the normal cell is reproducing or by something in the environment. Sometimes the cause of the DNA damage is something obvious, such as cigarette smoking. Often, however, no clear cause is found.

In most cases, the cancer cells form a **tumor**. Some cancers, such as leukemia, rarely form tumors. Instead, these cancer cells involve the blood and blood-forming organs and circulate through other tissues where they grow.

Cancer cells often travel to other parts of the body, where they begin to grow and form new tumors that replace normal tissue. This process is called **metastasis**. It happens when the cancer cells get into the bloodstream or lymph vessels of the body.

No matter where a cancer may spread, it is always named for the place where it started. For example, breast cancer that has spread to the liver is still called breast cancer, not liver cancer. Likewise, prostate cancer that has spread to the bone is **metastatic** prostate cancer, not bone cancer.

Different types of cancer can behave very differently. For example, lung cancer and breast cancer are very different diseases. They grow at different rates and respond to different treatments. That is why people with cancer need treatment that is aimed at their particular kind of cancer.

Not all tumors are cancerous. Tumors that are not cancer are called **benign**. Benign tumors can cause problems—they can grow very large and press on healthy organs and tissues. But they cannot grow into other tissues. Because they cannot invade other tissues, they also cannot **metastasize**, or spread, to other parts of the body. These tumors are almost never life threatening.

What Are Basal and Squamous Cell Skin Cancers?

To understand basal and squamous cell skin cancers, it helps to know about the normal structure and function of the skin.

Normal Skin

The skin is the largest organ in your body. It does several different things:

- covers the internal organs and protects them from injury
- serves as a barrier to germs such as bacteria
- prevents the loss of too much water and other fluids
- helps control body temperature

The skin has the following 3 layers:

- epidermis
- dermis
- subcutis

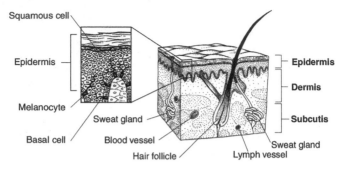

Epidermis

The top layer of skin is the **epidermis**. The epidermis is thin, averaging only 0.2 millimeters (mm) thick (about 1/100 of an inch). It protects the deeper layers of skin and the organs of the body from the environment.

Keratinocytes are the main cell type of the epidermis. These cells make an important protein called **keratin**, which gives the skin strength and flexibility and makes the skin waterproof.

The epidermis itself is made up of 3 sublayers. The outermost part of the epidermis is called the **stratum corneum**, or horny layer. It is composed of dead keratinocytes that are continually shed as new cells form. The cells in this layer are called **squamous cells** because of their flat shape.

Just below the stratum corneum are living keratinocytes. Below that is the **basal layer**, the inner layer of the epidermis. The cells of the basal layer, called **basal cells**, continually divide to form new keratinocytes. These new keratinocytes replace the older keratinocytes that slough off the skin's surface.

Cells called **melanocytes** are also present in the epidermis. These skin cells make the brown pigment called **melanin**. Melanin is what makes the skin tan or brown. It protects the deeper layers of the skin from some of the harmful effects of the sun.

The epidermis is separated from the deeper layers of skin by the **basement membrane**. The basement membrane is an important structure. When a skin cancer becomes more advanced, it generally grows through the basement membrane.

Dermis

The middle layer of the skin is called the **dermis**. The dermis is much thicker than the epidermis. It contains hair follicles, sweat glands, blood vessels, and nerves that are held in place by a protein called **collagen**. Collagen is made by cells called **fibroblasts** and gives the skin its resilience and strength.

Subcutis

The deepest layer of the skin is called the **subcutis**. The subcutis and the lowest part of the dermis form a network of collagen and fat cells. The subcutis helps the body conserve heat and has a shock-absorbing effect that helps protect the body's organs from injury.

Types of Skin Cancer

Melanomas

Cancers that develop from melanocytes, the pigment-making cells of the skin, are called

melanomas. Melanocytes can also form benign growths called **moles**. Melanoma and moles are discussed in the book *QuickFACTS™ Melanoma Skin Cancer*. Skin cancers that are not melanomas are sometimes grouped together as **nonmelanoma skin cancers** because they tend to act very differently from melanomas.

Keratinocyte cancers

Keratinocyte cancers are by far the largest group of nonmelanoma skin cancers. They are called **keratinocyte carcinomas** or keratinocyte cancers because, when seen under a microscope, their cells share some features of keratinocytes, the most abundant cell type of normal skin. The most common types of keratinocyte cancer are basal cell carcinoma and squamous cell carcinoma.

Basal Cell Carcinoma

Basal cell carcinoma is so named because the cells of these cancers resemble the cells in the lowest layer of epidermis, called the basal cell layer. About 8 out of 10 nonmelanoma skin cancers are basal cell carcinomas. They usually develop on sun-exposed areas, especially the head and neck. Basal cell carcinoma was once found almost exclusively in middle-aged or older adults. Now it is also being seen in younger adults, probably because they are spending more time in the sun with their skin exposed.

Basal cell carcinoma tends to be slow growing. It is very rare for a basal cell carcinoma to spread to lymph nodes or to distant parts of the body.

However, if a basal cell carcinoma is left untreated, it can grow into nearby areas and invade the bone or other tissues beneath the skin.

After treatment, basal cell carcinoma can recur (come back) in the same place on the skin. People who have had basal cell carcinoma are also more likely to get new ones elsewhere on the skin. In as many as half of people who have one basal cell carcinoma, a new basal cell skin cancer will develop within 5 years.

Squamous Cell Carcinoma

About 2 out of 10 nonmelanoma skin cancers are **squamous cell carcinomas**. They commonly appear on sun-exposed areas of the body, such as the face, ears, neck, lips, and back of the hands. They can also develop in scars or skin ulcers. They sometimes start in actinic keratoses (described on page 11). Less often, they can form in the skin of the genital area.

Squamous cell carcinomas tend to be more aggressive than basal cell carcinomas. They are more likely to invade fatty tissues just beneath the skin and are more likely to spread to lymph nodes and/or distant parts of the body, although this is still uncommon.

Keratoacanthomas are fairly common growths that are found on sun-exposed skin. These tumors closely resemble squamous cell carcinomas, and many doctors consider them to be a type of squamous cell cancer. They typically appear as firm, round, flesh-colored or red papules that progress to smooth, shiny dome-shaped nodules.

Although they may start out growing quickly, their growth usually slows down. Many keratoacanthomas shrink or even go away on their own over time without any treatment. But some continue to grow, and a few may even spread to other parts of the body. Their growth is often hard to predict.

Less Common Types of Skin Cancer

In addition to melanoma and keratinocyte cancers, there are other much less common types of skin cancer. These cancers are also nonmelanoma skin cancers, but they are quite different from keratinocyte cancers and are treated differently, so it is useful to consider them separately.

Other nonmelanoma skin cancers include the following:

- Merkel cell carcinoma
- Kaposi sarcoma
- Cutaneous lymphoma
- Skin adnexal tumors
- Various types of sarcomas

Together, these types account for less than 1% of nonmelanoma skin cancers.

Merkel cell carcinoma

Merkel cell carcinoma is an uncommon type of skin cancer that develops from **neuroendocrine cells** (hormone-making cells that resemble nerve cells) in the skin. They are most often found on the head, neck, and arms but can start anywhere. These cancers are thought to be caused in part by sun exposure and partly by **Merkel cell polyomavirus (MCV)**, a common virus that usually causes no **symptoms**. In a small percentage of people with this infection, changes in the virus's DNA can lead to this form of cancer. About 8 out of 10 Merkel cell carcinomas are thought to be related to MCV infection.

Unlike basal cell and squamous cell carcinomas, Merkel cell carcinomas often come back after treatment and can spread to nearby lymph nodes. They can also spread to internal organs, which is uncommon for squamous cell carcinomas and even less common for basal cell carcinomas. Treatment of Merkel cell carcinoma is described in the section "How Are Basal and Squamous Cell Skin Cancers Treated?"

Kaposi sarcoma

Kaposi sarcoma usually starts within the dermis but can also form in internal organs. Before the mid-1980s, this cancer was rare and found mostly in elderly people of Mediterranean descent. Kaposi sarcoma has become more common because it is more likely to develop in people with **human immunodeficiency virus (HIV)** infection and **acquired immunodeficiency syndrome (AIDS)**. For more information about Kaposi sarcoma, contact your American Cancer Society at **800-227-2345** and request the document *Kaposi Sarcoma* or visit our Web site, **cancer.org**.

Cutaneous lymphoma

Lymphomas are cancers that start in **lymphocytes**, a type of immune system cell. These immune system cells can be found in the **bone marrow**

(the soft inner part of some bones), **lymph nodes** (bean-sized collections of immune system cells), the bloodstream, and some internal organs. The skin also contains a significant number of lymphocytes.

Although most lymphomas start in lymph nodes or internal organs, there are certain types of lymphoma that appear to begin mostly or entirely in the skin. **Primary cutaneous lymphoma** means "a lymphoma that starts in the skin." The most common type of primary cutaneous lymphoma is **cutaneous T-cell lymphoma (CTCL)**. The most common type of CTCL is called **mycosis fungoides**. To learn more about cutaneous lymphoma, contact your American Cancer Society at **800-227-2345** to request the document *Lymphoma of the Skin* or visit our Web site, **cancer.org**.

Adnexal tumors

Adnexal tumors start in the hair follicles or glands (such as sweat glands) of the skin. **Malignant** (cancerous) adnexal tumors are rare, but benign (noncancerous) adnexal tumors are common.

Sarcomas

Sarcomas develop from connective tissue cells, usually in tissues deep beneath the skin. Much less often, they can develop in the skin's dermis and subcutis. Several types of sarcoma can develop in the skin, including **dermatofibrosarcoma protuberans (DFSP)** and **angiosarcoma** (a blood vessel cancer).

Precancerous and Preinvasive Skin Conditions

These conditions can develop into skin cancer or can be very early stages in the development of skin cancer.

Actinic keratosis (solar keratosis)

Actinic keratosis, also known as **solar keratosis**, is a precancerous skin condition caused by overexposure to the sun. Actinic keratoses are usually small (less than ¼ inch across), rough pinkish-red or flesh-colored spots. They are most common in middle-aged or older adults with fair skin and usually develop on the face, ears, back of the hands, and arms, although they can develop on other parts of the body that have been exposed to the sun. A person with one actinic keratosis usually develops many more.

Actinic keratoses are slow growing and usually do not cause any symptoms. It is possible for actinic keratoses to turn into keratinocyte cancers. Actinic keratoses often go away on their own, but they may come back.

Even though most actinic keratoses do not become cancers, they are a warning that your skin has suffered sun damage. Some actinic keratoses and other skin conditions that could be precancerous should be removed. Your doctor should regularly check any unusual or suspicious areas of skin for changes that could indicate cancer.

Squamous cell carcinoma in situ (Bowen disease)

Squamous cell carcinoma in situ, also called **Bowen disease**, is the earliest form of squamous cell skin cancer. "**In situ**" means that the cells of these cancers are still entirely within the epidermis and have not invaded the dermis.

Bowen disease appears as reddish patches. Compared with actinic keratoses, Bowen disease patches tend to be larger (sometimes more than ½ inch across), red, scaly, and sometimes crusted.

As with invasive squamous cell skin cancers, the main risk factor for Bowen disease is overexposure to the sun. Bowen disease of the anal and genital skin is often related to sexually transmitted infection with human papilloma viruses (HPVs), the viruses that can cause genital warts.

Benign Skin Tumors

Most tumors, or growths, of the skin are not cancerous and rarely, if ever, turn into cancers. These benign types of skin tumors include the following:

- most types of moles
- **seborrheic keratoses** (tan, brown, or black raised spots with a waxy texture or rough surface)
- **hemangiomas** (benign blood vessel growths often called strawberry spots or port wine stains)
- **lipomas** (soft growths of benign fat cells)
- **warts** (rough-surfaced growths caused by a virus)

What Are the Key Statistics About Basal and Squamous Cell Skin Cancers?

Cancer of the skin (including melanoma and basal and squamous cell skin cancers) is by far the most common of all types of cancer.

The number of people who develop basal and squamous cell skin cancers each year is not known for sure. Statistics of most other cancers are known because they are reported to cancer registries, but basal and squamous cell skin cancers are not reported. All the numbers presented here, therefore, are estimates.

About 2.2 million basal and squamous cell skin cancers are diagnosed each year. Most of these are basal cell cancers. Squamous cell cancers occur less often.

The number of these cancer diagnoses has been increasing for many years. This increase is probably due to a combination of increased detection, more sun exposure, and people living longer.

Death from these cancers is uncommon. It is thought that about 2,000 people die of nonmelanoma skin cancers each year. The death rate has dropped about 30% in the past 30 years. Most people who die are elderly. Other people more likely to die of skin cancer are those whose immune system is suppressed, such as people who have received organ transplants.

Risk Factors and Causes

What Are the Risk Factors for Basal and Squamous Cell Skin Cancers?

A **risk factor** is anything that affects your chance of a disease developing, such as cancer. Different types of cancer have different risk factors. For example, unprotected exposure to strong sunlight is a risk factor for skin cancer, and smoking is a risk factor for cancers of the lung, mouth, throat, kidneys, bladder, and several other organs.

Risk factors do not tell us everything, however. Having a risk factor, or even several risk factors, does not mean that you will get the disease. Many people who do not have any known risk factors still have skin cancer. Even if a person with basal or squamous cell skin cancer has a risk factor, it can be difficult to know how much that risk factor may have contributed to the cancer.

The following are known risk factors for basal cell and squamous cell carcinomas. (These factors do not necessarily apply to other forms of non-melanoma skin cancer, such as Kaposi sarcoma and cutaneous lymphoma.)

Exposure to Ultraviolet Radiation

Exposure to **ultraviolet (UV) radiation** is thought to be the main risk factor for most skin cancers. Sunlight is the main source of UV radiation, which can damage the **genes** in your skin cells. Tanning lamps, beds, and booths are another source of UV radiation. People with high levels of exposure to radiation from these sources are at greater risk for skin cancer.

Ultraviolet radiation is divided into 3 wavelength ranges:

- **UVA rays** cause cells to age and can cause some damage to cells' DNA. They are mainly linked to long-term skin damage such as wrinkles, but they are also thought to play a role in some skin cancers.
- **UVB rays** can cause direct damage to the DNA, and they are the rays that primarily cause sunburns. They are also thought to cause most skin cancers.
- **UVC rays** do not penetrate our atmosphere. They are not a cause of skin cancer.

Although UVA and UVB rays make up only a small portion of the sun's wavelengths, they are the main cause of the sun's damaging effects on the skin. UV radiation damages the DNA of skin cells. Skin cancers begin when this damage affects the DNA of genes that control skin cell growth. Both UVA and UVB rays damage skin and cause skin cancer. UVB rays are a more potent cause of at least some skin cancers, but based on what is known today, there are *no* safe UV rays.

The amount of exposure to UV radiation depends on the intensity of the radiation, the length of time the skin was exposed, and whether the skin was protected with clothing or sunscreen.

People who live in areas with year-round, bright sunlight are at higher risk for skin cancer. For example, the risk of skin cancer is twice as high in Arizona as in Minnesota. The highest rate of skin cancer in the world is in Australia. Spending a lot of time outdoors for work or recreation without protective clothing and sunscreen increases a person's risk of skin cancer.

Many studies also point to exposure at a young age (for example, frequent sunburns during childhood) as an added risk factor.

Fair Skin

The risk of skin cancer is much higher for whites than for blacks or Hispanics. This increased risk is caused by the protective effect of melanin in people with darker skin. Whites with fair skin that freckles or burns easily are at especially high risk. This factor is another reason for the high skin cancer rate in Australia, where much of the population is descended from fair-skinned immigrants from the British Isles.

Albinism is a **congenital** (present at birth) absence of skin pigment. People with this condition may have pinkish-white skin and white hair. They are at high risk of skin cancer unless they are careful to protect their skin from sun exposure.

Older Age

The risk of basal and squamous cell skin cancers goes up as people get older. This increase is probably due to accumulated sun exposure over time.

Male Gender

Men are about twice as likely as women to have basal cell cancers and about 3 times as likely to have squamous cell cancers of the skin. Increased levels of sun exposure is most likely the cause of this disparity between men and women.

Exposure to Certain Chemicals

Exposure to large amounts of arsenic increases the risk of skin cancer. Arsenic is a heavy metal found naturally in well water in some areas. It is also used in making some pesticides.

Workers exposed to industrial tar, coal, paraffin, and certain types of oil may also be at increased risk for nonmelanoma skin cancer.

Radiation Exposure

People who have had radiation therapy are at higher risk for skin cancer in the area that was treated. This is particularly a concern in children who have had radiation therapy for cancer.

Previous Skin Cancer

Anyone who has had a keratinocyte cancer has a much higher chance of another one developing.

Long-term or Severe Skin Inflammation or Injury

Scars from severe burns, areas of skin over severe bone infections, and skin damaged by some severe inflammatory skin diseases are more likely to develop keratinocyte skin cancers, although this risk is generally small.

Psoriasis Treatment

Psoralen and UVA radiation treatments (PUVA) given to some people with **psoriasis** (a long-lasting inflammatory skin disease) can increase the risk of squamous cell skin cancer and other skin cancers.

Xeroderma Pigmentosum

Xeroderma pigmentosum (XP) is a rare inherited condition that reduces the skin's ability to repair damage to DNA caused by sun exposure. People with this disorder often have many skin cancers, usually starting in childhood.

Basal Cell Nevus Syndrome

Basal cell nevus syndrome is a rare congenital (present at birth) condition that causes multiple basal cell cancers. In most cases, the condition is inherited. People with this syndrome may also have abnormalities of the jaw and other bones, eyes, and nervous tissue. In basal cell nevus syndrome, basal cell cancers often begin developing before the person reaches the age of 20.

Reduced Immunity

The immune system helps the body fight cancer. People whose immune systems have been weakened by certain diseases or medical treatments are more likely to have nonmelanoma skin cancer, particularly squamous cell cancer.

For example, people who undergo organ transplants are usually given medicines that weaken their immune systems to prevent their bodies from rejecting the new organ. The weakening of the immune system increases the risk of skin cancer. The rate of skin cancer in people who have had transplants can be as high as 70% in the 20 years following the transplant. Skin cancers in people with weakened immune systems tend to grow faster and are more likely to be fatal.

Treatment with large doses of corticosteroid drugs can also depress the immune system, which can increase a person's risk of skin cancer.

Human Papilloma Virus Infection

Human papilloma viruses (HPVs) are a group of more than 100 viruses that can cause **papillomas**, or warts. The warts that people commonly get on their hands and feet appear to be unrelated to any form of cancer. But some HPV types, especially those that cause warts in the genital and anal area, appear to be related to skin cancers in these areas.

Smoking

People who smoke are at higher risk for squamous cell skin cancer, especially on the lips. Smoking is not a known risk factor for basal cell skin cancer.

Do We Know What Causes Basal and Squamous Cell Skin Cancers?

Most basal cell and squamous cell skin cancers are caused by unprotected exposure to UV radiation.

This radiation comes from sunlight, as well as from man-made sources such as tanning booths.

Repeated and unprotected sun exposure over many years increases a person's risk of skin cancer. Most skin cancers are probably caused by exposure that happened many years earlier. The pattern of exposure may also be important. For example, frequent sunburns in childhood may increase the risk of basal cell skin cancer many years or even decades later.

DNA is the chemical in each of our cells that makes up our genes—the instructions for how our cells function. We usually look like our parents because they are the source of our DNA. However, DNA affects more than just how we look. Some genes contain instructions for controlling when our cells grow, divide, and die.

Exposure to UV radiation (from sunlight or tanning lamps) can damage DNA. Sometimes this damage affects certain genes that control how and when cells grow and divide. The cells can usually repair the damage, but in some cases the damage results in abnormal or mutated DNA, which may be the first step on the path to cancer.

Researchers do not yet know all of the DNA changes that result in skin cancer, but they have found that many skin cancers have mutated **tumor suppressor genes**. These genes normally function to help keep cells from growing out of control.

The gene most often found to be altered in squamous cell cancers is called **p53**. This gene normally causes damaged cells to die. When this gene is mutated, these abnormal cells may live longer and perhaps go on to become cancerous.

A gene commonly found to be mutated in basal cell cancers is the "patched" (*PTCH*) gene. This tumor suppressor gene normally helps keep cell growth in check, so changes in this gene can allow cells to grow out of control.

These are not the only gene changes that may play a role in the development of skin cancer. There are likely to be many others.

People with xeroderma pigmentosum (XP) are at high risk for skin cancer. XP is a rare, inherited condition that results from a defect in an enzyme that repairs damaged DNA. Because people with XP are less able to repair DNA damage caused by exposure to UV radiation, they develop huge numbers of cancers on sun-exposed areas of their skin.

The link between squamous cell skin cancer and human papilloma virus (HPV) infection also involves DNA and genes. These viruses contain genes that instruct infected cells to make proteins that affect the growth of skin cells. These proteins can cause skin cells to grow too much and not die when they should.

Scientists are studying other links between DNA changes and skin cancer. In the future, better understanding of how damaged DNA leads to skin cancer might be used to design treatments to overcome or repair that damage.

Prevention and Detection

Can Basal and Squamous Cell Skin Cancers Be Prevented?

While not all basal and squamous cell skin cancers can be prevented, there are ways to reduce your risk of skin cancer.

Limit Exposure to Ultraviolet Radiation

The most important way to lower your risk of basal and squamous cell skin cancers is to limit your exposure to ultraviolet (UV) radiation. Practice sun safety when you are outdoors. "Slip! Slop! Slap! . . . and Wrap" is a catch phrase that can help you remember the 4 key methods you can use to protect yourself from UV radiation:

- Slip on a shirt.
- Slop on sunscreen.
- Slap on a hat.
- Wrap on sunglasses to protect the eyes and sensitive skin around them.

Protect your skin with clothing

Clothes provide different levels of UV protection, depending on many factors. Long-sleeved shirts, long pants, or long skirts are the most protective. Dark colors generally provide more protection than light colors. Tightly woven fabrics protect better than loosely woven fabrics. Dry fabric is generally more protective than wet fabric.

Be aware that covering up does not block out all UV radiation. If you can see light through a fabric, UV radiation can get through, too.

Some companies in the United States now make clothing that is lightweight, comfortable, and protects against exposure to UV radiation even when wet. These sun-protective clothes may have a label listing the **ultraviolet protection factor (UPF)** value—the level of protection the garment provides from the sun's UV rays (on a scale from 15 to 50+). The higher the UPF, the higher the protection from UV radiation.

Newer products, which are used in the washing machine in the same way as detergent, can increase the UPF value of clothes you already own. These products add a layer of UV protection to your clothes without changing the color or texture.

Wear a hat

A hat with at least a 2- to 3-inch brim all around is ideal because it protects areas often exposed to intense sun, such as the ears, eyes, forehead, nose, and scalp. A shade cap also protects these sensitive areas. Often sold in sporting goods and outdoor supply stores, a shade cap looks like a baseball cap with about 7 inches of fabric draping down the sides and back. A baseball cap can protect the front and top of the head but not the neck or the ears, where skin cancers commonly develop. Straw hats are not as protective as ones made of tightly woven fabric.

Use sunscreen

Use sunscreens and lip balms on areas of skin exposed to the sun, especially when the sunlight is strong (for example, in hot or high-altitude locations and between the hours of 10 A.M. and 4 P.M.). Many groups, including the American Academy of Dermatology, recommend using products with a **sun protection factor (SPF)** of 30 or more. Use sunscreen even on hazy days or days with light or broken cloud cover because the UV radiation still comes through.

Always follow directions when applying sunscreen. For an average adult, a 1-ounce application (about 2 tablespoons) is recommended to cover the arms, legs, neck, and face. Protection is greatest when sunscreen is applied thickly on all sun-exposed skin. To ensure continued protection, sunscreens should be reapplied; it is often recommended to do so every 2 hours. Many sunscreens wash off when you sweat or swim or can be wiped off by toweling dry, so they must be reapplied for maximum effectiveness. Do not forget your lips; lip balm with sunscreen is also available.

According to new labeling rules by the **U.S. Food and Drug Administration (FDA)**, only sunscreens that protect against both UVA and UVB rays may be labeled as "broad spectrum." The new FDA rules also state that only sunscreens that are both broad spectrum and have an SPF of 15 or higher may state that they reduce the risk of skin cancer and early skin aging, when used as directed. These labeling rules are expected to become effective in 2012.

Some people use sunscreen so they can stay out in the sun longer without getting sunburned. Sunscreen should not be used to gain extra time in the sun, because you will still end up with damage to your skin. Sunscreen can reduce your risk of actinic keratoses and squamous cell cancer. There is no guarantee, however, and if you stay in the sun a long time, you are at risk for skin cancer even if you have applied sunscreen.

If you want a tan, try using a sunless tanning lotion. These products can provide the desired look without the danger. Sunless tanning lotions contain a substance called **dihydroxyacetone (DHA)**. DHA works by interacting with proteins on the surface of the skin to produce color. You do not have to be in the sun for these products to work. The color tends to wear off after a few days.

Wear sunglasses

Wrap-around sunglasses with at least 99% UV absorption provide the best protection for your eyes and the skin around your eyes. Look for sunglasses labeled as blocking UVA and UVB rays. Labels that say "UV absorption up to 400 nm" or "Meets ANSI UV Requirements" mean the glasses block at least 99% of UV rays. If there is no label, do not assume the sunglasses provide any protection.

Seek shade

Another way to limit exposure to UV radiation is to avoid being outdoors in sunlight too long. This is particularly important in the middle of the day between the hours of 10 A.M. and 4 P.M., when UV radiation is strongest. If you are unsure about the sun's intensity, use the shadow test: if your shadow is shorter than you, the sun's rays are at their strongest, and it is important to protect yourself.

When you are outdoors, protect your skin. Keep in mind that sunlight (and UV radiation) can come through light clouds; can reflect off water, sand, concrete, and snow; and can reach below the water's surface.

The UV Index: The amount of UV radiation reaching the ground in any given place depends on a number of factors, including the time of day, time of year, elevation, and cloud cover. To help people better understand the intensity of UV radiation in their area on a given day, the National Weather Service and the Environmental Protection Agency have developed the **UV Index**. This number gives people an idea of the strength of the UV radiation in their area, on a scale from 1 (low) to 11+ (extremely high). A higher number means a higher chance of sunburn, skin damage, and ultimately skin cancers of all kinds. Your local UV Index should be available daily in your local newspaper, on television weather reports, and on the Web site www.epa.gov/sunwise/uvindex.html.

Avoid Tanning Beds and Sunlamps

Many people believe the UV rays of tanning beds are harmless. This is not true. Tanning lamps give out UVA and usually UVB rays as well, both of which can cause long-term skin damage and can contribute to skin cancer. Most dermatologists and health organizations recommend not using tanning beds and sunlamps.

Protect Children from the Sun

Children need special attention because they tend to spend more time outdoors and can burn more easily. Parents and other caregivers should protect children from sun exposure by using the measures already described. Older children need to be cautioned about sun exposure as they become more independent. It is important, particularly in parts of the world where it is sunnier, to cover your children as fully as is reasonable. You should develop the habit of using sunscreen on exposed skin for yourself and your children whenever you go outdoors and may be exposed to large amounts of sunlight.

Children's swimsuits made from sun-protective fabric and designed to cover the child from the neck to the knees are popular in Australia. They are now available in the United States. Babies younger than 6 months should be kept out of direct sunlight and protected from the sun by using hats and protective clothing.

Sun Exposure and Vitamin D

Doctors are learning that **vitamin D** has many health benefits. It may even help to lower the risk of some cancers. Vitamin D is made naturally by your skin when you are exposed to sunlight. How much vitamin D you get depends on many things, including how old you are, how dark your skin is, and how intensely the sun shines where you live.

At this time, doctors are not sure of the optimal level of vitamin D. A lot of research is being done in this area. It is better to get vitamin D from your diet or vitamin supplements than from sun exposure, because dietary sources and vitamin supplements do not increase risk of skin cancer and are typically more reliable ways to get the amount you need.

For more information on how to protect yourself and your family from exposure to UV radiation, contact your American Cancer Society at **800-227-2345** to request the document *Skin Cancer Prevention and Early Detection* or visit our Web site, **cancer.org**.

Avoid Harmful Chemicals

Exposure to certain chemicals, such as **arsenic**, can increase a person's risk of skin cancer. People can be exposed to arsenic from well water in some areas, pesticides and herbicides, some medicines (such as arsenic trioxide) and herbal remedies (arsenic was found in some traditional herbal remedies imported from China), and in certain occupations (such as mining and smelting).

Learn More About Skin Cancer Prevention

Many organizations conduct skin cancer prevention activities in schools and recreational areas. Others provide brochures and public service announcements. For more information, see the "Resources" section on page 81.

Can Basal and Squamous Cell Skin Cancers Be Found Early?

Basal cell and squamous cell skin cancers can be found early. As part of a routine cancer-related checkup, your health care professional should check your skin carefully. He or she should be willing to discuss any doubts or concerns you might have about this examination.

You can also play an important role in finding skin cancer early. It is important to check your skin thoroughly, preferably once a month. Learn the patterns of moles, blemishes, freckles, and other marks on your skin so that you will notice any changes. Self-examinations are best done in a well-lit room in front of a full-length mirror. A hand-held mirror can be used for areas that are hard to see.

Examine all areas of your body, including your palms and the soles of your feet, your scalp, ears, nails, and your back. Friends and family members can also help you with these exams, especially for hard-to-see areas, such as your lower back or the back of your thighs. Be sure to show your doctor any area that concerns you. For a more thorough description of a skin self-examination, contact your American Cancer Society at **800-227-2345** and request the documents *Skin Cancer Prevention and Early Detection* and *Why You Should Know About Melanoma* or visit our Web site, **cancer.org**.

Spots on the skin that are new or changing in size, shape, or color should be evaluated promptly. Any unusual sore, lump, blemish, marking, or change in the way an area of the skin looks or feels may be a **sign** of skin cancer or a warning that it might occur. The skin might become scaly or crusty or begin oozing or bleeding. It may feel itchy, tender, or painful. Redness and swelling may develop. Spots on the skin that look different from the surrounding moles should be evaluated.

Basal cell and squamous cell skin cancers can look like a variety of marks on the skin. The key warning signs are a new growth, a spot or bump that is getting larger (over a few months or 1 to 2 years), or a sore that does not heal within 2 months. For a more detailed description of what to look for, see the next section, "How Are Basal and Squamous Cell Skin Cancers Diagnosed?"

Diagnosis and Staging

How Are Basal and Squamous Cell Skin Cancers Diagnosed?

If an abnormal area of skin indicates the possibility of skin cancer, certain medical examinations and tests such as a **biopsy** may be used to find out whether it is cancer or some other skin condition. If there is a chance the skin cancer may have spread to other areas of the body, other tests may be done as well.

Signs and Symptoms of Basal and Squamous Cell Skin Cancers

Skin cancers rarely cause bothersome symptoms until they become quite large. Then they may bleed or even hurt.

Basal cell carcinomas often appear as flat, firm, pale areas or raised pink or red, translucent, shiny, waxy areas. The area may bleed easily. They may have one or more visible abnormal blood vessels and/or blue, brown, or black areas. Large basal cell carcinomas may have oozing or crusted areas. They usually develop on areas exposed to the sun, especially the head and neck, but they can occur anywhere on the body.

Squamous cell carcinomas may appear as growing lumps, often with a rough, scaly, or crusted surface. They may also appear as flat reddish patches on the skin that grow slowly. They commonly occur on sun-exposed areas of the body such as the face, ears, neck, lips, and back of the hands. Less often, they form on the skin of the genital area. They can also develop on scars or skin ulcers elsewhere on the body.

Both basal cell and squamous cell skin cancers can develop as flat areas showing only slight changes from normal skin.

Skin cancers other than melanoma, basal cell carcinoma, and squamous cell carcinoma are much less common and may look different.

- **Kaposi sarcoma** generally starts as a small bruise-like area that develops into a reddish or purplish tumor under the skin.
- **Mycosis fungoides** (a type of lymphoma that starts in the skin) usually begins as a rash, often on the buttocks, hips, or lower abdomen. It can look like a skin allergy or other type of skin irritation.
- **Adnexal tumors** appear as bumps within the skin.
- **Skin sarcomas** appear as large masses under the surface of the skin.
- **Merkel cell tumors** are usually firm pink, red, or purple nodules or ulcers found on the face or, less often, the arms or legs.

If your doctor suspects you might have skin cancer, he or she will use one or more of the following methods to diagnose the condition.

Medical History and Physical Examination

Usually the doctor's first step will be to take your medical history. The doctor probably will ask your age, when the mark on the skin first appeared, and whether it has changed in size or appearance. You may also be asked about past exposures to known causes of skin cancer (including sunburns) and whether you or anyone in your family has had skin cancer.

During the physical examination, the doctor will note the size, shape, color, and texture of the area(s) in question, and whether there is bleeding or scaling. The rest of your body may be checked for spots and moles that could be related to skin cancer.

The doctor may also check nearby lymph nodes. Some skin cancers may spread to lymph nodes. When this happens, the lymph nodes may become larger and firmer than usual.

If you are being seen by your primary care doctor and skin cancer is suspected, you may be referred to a dermatologist (a doctor who specializes in skin diseases) who will examine the area more closely.

Along with a standard physical examination, some dermatologists use a technique called **dermatoscopy** (also known as dermoscopy, **epiluminescence microscopy [ELM]**, or surface microscopy) to see spots on the skin more clearly. The doctor uses a dermatoscope, which is a special magnifying lens and light source held near the skin. A digital or photographic image of the spot may be taken.

When performed by an experienced dermatologist, this test can improve the accuracy of finding skin cancers early. Often, it can reassure you that a lesion is benign without the need for a biopsy.

Skin Biopsy

If the doctor thinks that a suspicious area might be skin cancer, he or she will take a sample of skin from the area to be looked at under a microscope. This procedure is called a **skin biopsy**. Different methods can be used for a skin biopsy. The choice depends on what type of skin cancer is suspected, its location on your body, the size of the affected area, and other factors. Any biopsy is likely to leave a scar. Because different methods produce different scars, you should ask your doctor about scarring before the biopsy is done if you are concerned.

Shave biopsy

A **shave biopsy** is one way to take a skin biopsy. After numbing the area with a local **anesthetic**, the doctor shaves off the top layers of the skin (the epidermis and the most superficial part of the dermis) with a surgical blade.

Punch biopsy

A **punch biopsy** removes a deeper sample of skin. The doctor uses a tool that looks like a tiny round cookie cutter. Once the skin is numbed with a local anesthetic, the doctor rotates the punch biopsy tool on the surface of the skin until it cuts through all the layers of the skin, including the dermis, epidermis, and the upper parts of the subcutis.

Incisional and excisional biopsies

If the doctor has to examine a tumor that may have grown into deeper layers of the skin, he or she will use an incisional or excisional biopsy technique. An **incisional biopsy** removes only a portion of the tumor, whereas an **excisional biopsy** removes the entire tumor. A surgical knife is used to cut through the full thickness of skin. A wedge or sliver of skin is removed for examination, and the edges of the wound are sewn together. Both of these types of biopsies can usually be done with **local anesthesia** to numb the area first.

Examining the Biopsy Samples

All skin biopsy samples will be looked at under a microscope by a pathologist, a doctor who has been specially trained in the examination and **diagnosis** of tissue samples. Often, the sample is sent to a dermatopathologist, a doctor who has special training in making diagnoses from skin samples.

Lymph Node Biopsy

If your doctor feels lymph nodes that are too large or too firm, a lymph node biopsy may be done to determine whether cancer has spread from the skin to the lymph nodes.

Fine needle aspiration biopsy

A **fine needle aspiration (FNA) biopsy** uses a syringe with a thin, hollow needle to remove very small tissue fragments from a tumor. The needle is smaller than the needle used for a blood test. A local anesthetic is sometimes used to numb the area first. This test rarely causes much discomfort and does not leave a scar.

An FNA biopsy is not used to diagnose a suspicious skin tumor, but it may be used to biopsy lymph nodes near a skin cancer to find out whether the cancer has spread to them.

Surgical (excisional) lymph node biopsy

If the doctor suspects cancer has spread to a lymph node but the FNA result is negative or unclear, the lymph node will be removed by surgery and examined. This procedure can often be done in a doctor's office or outpatient surgical center using local anesthesia and will leave a small scar.

How Are Basal and Squamous Cell Skin Cancers Staged?

The **stage** of cancer describes the extent of the cancer in the body. **Staging** is a process of finding out how far the cancer has spread. Because basal cell cancer so rarely spreads to other organs, it is seldom staged unless the cancer is very large. Squamous cell cancers have a somewhat greater (but still quite small) risk of spreading, so staging may sometimes be done, particularly in people who have a high risk of metastasis. This high-risk group includes people with suppressed immune systems, such as those who have had organ transplants and people who are HIV-positive.

The tests and examinations described in the section "How Are Basal and Squamous Cell Skin Cancers Diagnosed?" are the main ones used to help determine the stage of the cancer. In rare cases, imaging tests such as **x-rays**, **computed tomography (CT) scans**, or **MRI** scans may be used as well.

The American Joint Committee on Cancer (AJCC) TNM System

A staging system is a way to summarize how far a cancer has spread. This helps members of the **cancer care team** plan appropriate treatment and determine a person's **prognosis** (outlook).

The system most often used to stage keratinocyte cancers (especially squamous cell skin cancer) is the **American Joint Commission on Cancer (AJCC) TNM system.** (Merkel cell carcinoma has a separate AJCC staging system, which is not described here.)

Physical examinations and other tests may be used to assign T, N, and M categories and a grouped stage. The TNM system for staging contains the following 3 key pieces of information:

- **T** stands for **tumor** (its size, location, and how far it has spread within the skin and to nearby tissues).
- **N** stands for spread to nearby lymph **nodes**.
- **M** is for **metastasis** (spread to distant organs).

T categories

The possible values for T are as follows:

- **TX:** Primary tumor cannot be assessed.
- **T0:** No evidence of primary tumor.
- **Tis:** Carcinoma in situ (tumor is still confined to the epidermis).
- **T1:** Tumor is 2 centimeters (cm) across (about ⅘ inch) or smaller and has no more than 1 high-risk feature (see page 40).

- **T2:** Tumor is larger than 2 cm across or has 2 or more high-risk features.
- **T3:** Tumor invades facial bones, such as the jaw bones or bones around the eye.
- **T4:** Tumor invades other bones in the body or the base of the skull.

High-risk features: These features are used to distinguish between some T1 and T2 tumors.

- Tumor is thicker than 2 millimeters (mm).
- Tumor has invaded the lower dermis or subcutis (Clark level IV or V).
- Tumor has invaded tiny nerves in the skin (perineural invasion).
- Tumor started on an ear or on a hair-bearing lip.
- Tumor cells look very abnormal (poorly differentiated or undifferentiated) when viewed under a microscope.

N categories

The possible values for N are as follows:

NX: Nearby lymph nodes cannot be assessed.

N0: No spread to nearby lymph nodes.

N1: Spread to 1 nearby lymph node that is on the same side of the body as the main tumor and is 3 cm or less across.

N2a: Spread to 1 nearby lymph node that is on the same side of the body as the main tumor and is between 3 and 6 cm across.

N2b: Spread to more than 1 nearby lymph node on the same side of the body as the main tumor. None of the lymph nodes are larger than 6 cm across.

N2c: Spread to nearby lymph node(s) on the other side of the body from the main tumor. None of the lymph nodes are larger than 6 cm across.

N3: Spread to any nearby lymph node that is larger than 6 cm across.

M categories

The M values are as follows:

MX: Presence of distant metastasis cannot be assessed.

M0: No spread to distant organs.

M1: Spread to distant organs.

Stage Grouping

To assign a stage, information about the tumor and whether it has spread to lymph nodes and other organs in the body is combined in a process called stage grouping. The stages are described by using the number 0 and Roman numerals from I to IV. In general, people with lower-stage cancers tend to have a better prognosis for a cure or long-term survival.

Stage Grouping Based on T, N, and M Values

Stage 0	Tis, N0, M0
Stage I	T1, N0, M0
Stage II	T2, N0, M0
Stage III	T3, N0, M0 T1 to T3, N1, M0
Stage IV	T1 to T3, N2, M0 Any T, N3, M0 T4, any N, M0 Any T, any N, M1

Treatment

How Are Basal and Squamous Cell Skin Cancers Treated?

Most basal cell and squamous cell cancers can be completely cured by fairly minor surgery or other types of local treatments. The treatments described in this section may be used for actinic keratosis, squamous cell carcinoma, basal cell carcinoma, and Merkel cell carcinoma. Lymphoma of the skin, Kaposi sarcoma, and other sarcomas are treated differently and are not discussed in this book. For more information about treatments for these skin conditions, contact your American Cancer Society at **800-227-2345** or visit our Web site, **cancer.org**.

Surgery

There are many different kinds of surgery for basal cell and squamous cell skin cancers. The type of treatment chosen depends on the cancer's size, its location on the body, and the type of skin cancer. For certain squamous cell cancers with a high risk of spreading, surgery may sometimes be followed by radiation or chemotherapy.

Simple excision

This procedure is similar to an excisional biopsy. For this procedure, the skin is first numbed with a local anesthetic. The tumor is then cut out with a surgical knife, along with some surrounding normal skin. The remaining skin is carefully stitched back together, leaving a small scar.

Shave excision

In a shave excision, the abnormal area is shaved off the skin's surface by using a small blade.

Curettage and electrodesiccation

Curettage and electrodesiccation removes the cancer by scraping it with a **curette** (a long, thin instrument with a sharp edge on one end). A needle-shaped electrode is then used to treat the area with an electric current to destroy any remaining cancer cells. This process is often repeated several times during the surgery to remove all of the cancer. Curettage and electrodesiccation is often recommended for small basal cell and squamous cell cancers. It will leave a scar.

Mohs surgery (microscopically controlled surgery)

In Mohs surgery, the surgeon cuts the tumor from the skin in thin layers, examining each sample under a microscope. If cancer cells are seen, deeper layers are removed and examined until the skin samples are found to be free of cancer cells. This process is slow, but it means that more normal skin near the tumor can be saved, which will create a better appearance after surgery. **Mohs surgery** is a highly specialized technique that should be used only by doctors who have been trained in this specific type of surgery.

Lymph node surgery

If lymph nodes near a nonmelanoma skin cancer (especially a squamous cell or Merkel cell carcinoma) are growing, doctors will want to determine whether the cancer has spread to these lymph nodes. The nodes may be biopsied or removed by a procedure called a lymph node dissection and examined under a microscope for signs of cancer. This procedure is more involved than surgery on the skin and usually requires general anesthesia (in which you are asleep).

Lymphedema, a complication in which excess fluid collects in the legs or arms, is a possible long-term side effect of a lymph node dissection. Lymph nodes in the groin or under the arms normally help drain fluid from the legs and arms. If the lymph nodes are removed, fluid may build up, leading to swelling in these limbs. Elastic stockings or compression sleeves can help some people with this condition. For more information about lymphedema, contact your American Cancer Society at **800-227-2345** and request the document *Understanding Lymphedema (For Cancers Other Than Breast Cancer)* or visit our Web site, **cancer.org**.

Skin grafting and reconstructive surgery

After removing large nonmelanoma skin cancers, it may not be possible to stretch the nearby skin enough to sew the edges of the wound together. In these cases, healthy skin may be taken from another part of the body and grafted over the wound to help it heal and to restore the appearance of the affected area. Other reconstructive surgical procedures can also be helpful in some cases.

Other Forms of Local Therapy

Several other techniques can be used to treat basal and squamous cell skin cancers that have not spread to lymph nodes or other parts of the body. Some of these treatments are described as surgery because they destroy a targeted area of body tissue. These techniques do not, however, involve using scalpels or cutting into the skin.

Cryosurgery (cryotherapy)

During **cryosurgery**, liquid nitrogen is applied to the tumor to freeze and kill abnormal cells. After the dead tissue thaws, blistering and crusting may occur. The wound can take 1 or 2 months to heal and will leave a scar. The treated area may have less color after treatment. Cryosurgery is often used for precancerous conditions such as actinic keratosis and for small basal cell and squamous cell carcinomas.

Photodynamic therapy

In **photodynamic therapy (PDT)**, a chemical is applied to the skin or injected into the blood. This chemical collects in the tumor cells over the course of several hours or days and makes the cells sensitive to certain types or colors of light. A light source is then focused on the tumor(s), which causes the cells to die. A possible side effect of PDT is that it can make the person's skin very sensitive to sunlight for a period of time (often several weeks), so precautions may be needed to avoid severe burns.

PDT can be used to treat actinic keratoses. Its role in treating nonmelanoma skin cancers, however, still needs to be determined.

Topical chemotherapy

Chemotherapy uses drugs to kill cancer cells. **Topical chemotherapy** means that an anticancer medicine is placed directly on the skin (usually in the form of a cream or ointment) rather than being given by mouth or injected into a vein. The drug most often used in topical treatment of basal and squamous cell skin cancers is **5-fluorouracil (5-FU)**.

When applied directly to the skin in cream form, 5-FU can reach cancer cells near the skin surface but cannot reach cancer cells that have invaded deeper skin tissues or spread to other organs. For this reason, 5-FU is used only for precancerous conditions such as actinic keratosis and for some superficial skin cancers.

Because it is applied to the skin only, the drug does not spread throughout the body, and therefore it does not cause the same side effects that can occur with systemic chemotherapy (treatment that affects the whole body). However, it can cause the treated skin to become red and very sensitive for a few weeks, which can be bothersome for some people. Other topical medicines can be used to help relieve this side effect. Fluorouracil also increases the skin's sensitivity to sunlight, so treated areas must be protected from the sun for a few weeks to prevent sunburn.

A gel containing the drug diclofenac is sometimes used to treat actinic keratoses. This drug is a **nonsteroidal anti-inflammatory drug (NSAID)**, a type of medication that includes pain relievers such as aspirin and ibuprofen.

Immune response modifiers

Certain drugs can boost the body's immune system response to the cancer, causing it to regress (get smaller and go away). These drugs are called **immune response modifiers**.

Imiquimod is a cream that can be applied to actinic keratoses and some basal cell cancers. It causes the immune system to react to the skin lesion and destroy it.

Interferon is a man-made version of an immune system protein. It can be injected directly into the tumor to boost the immune response against it. It is used occasionally in cases in which surgery is not possible, but it may not be as effective as other treatments.

Laser surgery

Laser surgery is a relatively new approach that uses a laser beam to vaporize cancer cells. It is sometimes used for squamous cell carcinoma in situ (involving only the epidermis) and for very superficial basal cell carcinomas (those located near the surface of the skin). It is not yet known whether this type of treatment is as effective as standard methods of treatment, and it is not widely used.

Radiation Therapy

Radiation therapy uses high-energy rays (such as x-rays) or particles (such as photons, electrons, or protons) to kill cancer cells. **External beam radiation therapy** focuses radiation from outside the body on the skin tumor. The treatment is much like getting an x-ray, but the radiation is more intense. The procedure itself is painless. Each treatment lasts only a few minutes, although the setup time—getting you into place for treatment—takes longer.

If a tumor is very large or is located on an area of the skin that makes surgery difficult, radiation may be used as the primary treatment instead of surgery. Using radiation therapy as the primary treatment can be useful for elderly people who cannot tolerate surgery because of poor general health. Radiation therapy can cure small nonmelanoma skin cancers and can slow the growth of more advanced cancers. Radiation is also useful in combination with other therapies. It is particularly useful for treating Merkel cell carcinoma.

In some cases, radiation can be used after surgery as **adjuvant therapy** (a term for any treatment after surgery) to kill any small deposits of remaining cancer cells that may not have been visible during surgery. Adjuvant therapy lowers the risk of cancer **recurrence**. Radiation may also be used to help treat nonmelanoma skin cancer that has spread to lymph nodes or other organs.

Side effects of radiation can include skin irritation, redness, and drying. With longer treatments, these side effects may get worse. After many years, new skin cancers can sometimes develop in areas previously treated by radiation. For this reason, radiation usually is not used to treat skin cancer in young people. Radiation is also not recommended for people with certain inherited conditions (such as basal cell nevus syndrome) because they may be more vulnerable to the cancer-causing side effects of radiation.

For more information about radiation therapy, please contact your American Cancer Society at **800-227-2345** and request the document *Understanding Radiation Therapy: A Guide for Patients and Families* or visit our Web site, **cancer.org**.

Systemic Chemotherapy

Systemic chemotherapy uses anticancer drugs that are injected into a vein or given by mouth. These drugs travel through the bloodstream to all parts of the body. In contrast to topical chemotherapy, systemic chemotherapy can attack cancer cells that have spread to lymph nodes and other organs.

One or more chemotherapy drugs may be used to treat squamous cell carcinoma or Merkel cell carcinoma that has spread to other organs. Chemotherapy drugs such as cisplatin, doxorubicin, 5-FU, and mitomycin are given intravenously (into a vein), usually once every few weeks. They can often delay the spread of these cancers and relieve some symptoms. In some cases, these drugs may shrink tumors enough that other treatments such as surgery or radiation therapy can be used.

Chemotherapy drugs work by attacking cells that are dividing quickly, which is why they work against cancer cells. Other cells in the body, however, such as those in the bone marrow, the lining of the mouth and intestines, and the hair follicles, also divide quickly. These cells are also likely to be affected by chemotherapy, which can lead to side effects.

The side effects of chemotherapy depend on the type and dose of drugs given and the length of time they are taken. These side effects may include the following:

- hair loss
- mouth sores
- loss of appetite
- nausea and vomiting
- lowered resistance to infection (because of low white blood cell counts)
- easy bruising or bleeding (because of low blood platelet counts)
- fatigue (because of low red blood cell counts)

These side effects are usually short term and go away once treatment is finished. There are often ways to lessen these side effects. For example, drugs can be given to help prevent or reduce nausea and vomiting. Do not hesitate to discuss side effects with the cancer care team. You should tell your medical team about any side effects or changes you notice while getting chemotherapy so that they can be treated promptly. For more general information about chemotherapy, please contact your American Cancer Society at **800-227-2345** and request the document *Understanding Chemotherapy: A Guide for Patients and Families* or visit our Web site: **cancer.org**.

Clinical Trials

If you have been told you have skin cancer, you have a lot of decisions to make. One of the most important decisions you will make is deciding which treatment is best for you. You may have heard about clinical trials being done for your type of cancer. Or maybe someone on your health care team has mentioned a **clinical trial** to you. Clinical trials are one way to get state-of-the art cancer care. Still, they are not right for everyone.

Here, we will give you a brief overview of clinical trials. Talking to your health care team, your family, and your friends can help you make the best treatment choices.

Clinical trials are carefully controlled research studies that are done with patients. These studies test whether a new treatment is safe and how well it works in patients, or they may test new ways to diagnose or prevent a disease. Clinical trials have led to many advances in cancer prevention, diagnosis, and treatment.

Clinical trials are done to get a closer look at promising new treatments or procedures in patients. A clinical trial is undertaken only when there is good reason to believe that the treatment, test, or procedure being studied may be better than the one already being used. Treatments used in clinical trials are often found to have real benefits and may go on to become tomorrow's standard treatment.

Clinical trials can focus on many things:

- new uses of drugs that are already approved by the U.S. Food and Drug Administration (FDA)

- new drugs that have not yet been approved by the FDA
- nondrug treatments (such as radiation therapy)
- medical procedures (such as types of surgery)
- herbs and vitamins
- tools to improve the ways medicines or diagnostic tests are used
- medicines or procedures to relieve symptoms or improve comfort
- combinations of treatments and procedures

Researchers conduct studies of new treatments to try to answer the following questions:

- Is the treatment helpful?
- What is the best way to give it?
- Does it work better than other treatments already available?
- What side effects does the treatment cause?
- Are there more or fewer side effects than the standard treatment used now?
- Do the benefits outweigh the side effects?
- In which patients is the treatment most likely to be helpful?

Clinical trials are usually conducted in distinct phases. Each phase is designed to answer certain questions. Knowing the phase of the clinical trial is important because it can give you some idea about how much is known about the treatment being studied. There are pros and cons to taking part in each phase of a clinical trial.

Phase 0 clinical trials

Even though phase 0 studies are done in humans, this type of study is not much like the other phases of clinical trials. It is included here because some cancer patients may be asked to take part in these kinds of studies in the future.

Phase 0 studies are exploratory studies that often use only a few small doses of a new drug in each patient. They test to find out whether the drug reaches the tumor, how the drug acts in the human body, and how cancer cells respond to the drug. The patients in these studies must have extra biopsies, scans, and blood samples. The biggest difference between phase 0 and the later phases of clinical trials is that there is no chance the patient will be helped by taking part in a phase 0 trial. Because drug doses are low, there is also less risk to the patient in phase 0 studies compared with phase I studies.

Phase 0 studies help researchers find out which drugs do not do what they are expected to do. If there are problems with the way the drug is absorbed or acts in the body, this should become clear very quickly in a phase 0 trial. This process may help avoid the delay and expense of finding out years later in phase II or even phase III clinical trials that the drug doesn't act as it was expected to, based on laboratory studies.

Phase 0 studies are not yet being used widely, and there are some drugs for which they would not be helpful. Phase 0 studies are very small, mostly with fewer than 20 people. They are not a required part of testing a new drug but are part of an effort to speed up and streamline the process.

Phase I clinical trials

The purpose of a phase I study is to find the safest way to give a new treatment to patients. The cancer care team closely watches patients for any harmful side effects.

For phase I studies, the drug has already been tested in laboratory and animal studies, but the side effects in patients are not fully known. Doctors start by giving very low doses of the drug to the first patients and increase the doses for later groups of patients until side effects appear or the desired effect is seen. Doctors are hoping to help the study patients, but the main purpose of a phase I trial is to test the safety of the drug.

Phase I clinical trials are often done in small groups of people with different cancers that have not responded to standard treatment or that recur after treatment. If a drug is found to be reasonably safe in phase I studies, it can be tested in a phase II clinical trial.

Phase II clinical trials

These studies are designed to see whether the drug is effective. Patients are given the most appropriate (safest) dose as determined from phase I studies. They are closely watched for an effect on the cancer. The cancer care team also looks for side effects. Phase II trials are often done in larger groups of patients with a specific cancer type that has not responded to standard treatment. If a drug is found to be effective in phase II studies, it can be tested in a phase III clinical trial.

Phase III clinical trials

Phase III studies involve large numbers of patients—most often those patients who have just received a diagnosis for a specific type of cancer. Phase III clinical trials may enroll thousands of patients. Often, these studies are randomized, which means that patients are randomly put in 1 of 2 (or more) groups. One group (called the **control group**) gets the standard, most accepted treatment. The other group(s) gets the new treatment(s) being studied. All patients in phase III studies are closely watched. The study will be stopped early if many patients experience side effects that are too severe or if one group has much better results than the others. Phase III clinical trials are needed before the FDA will approve a treatment for use by the general public.

Phase IV clinical trials

Once a drug has been approved by the FDA and is available for all patients, it is still studied in other clinical trials (sometimes referred to as phase IV studies). This way, more can be learned about short-term and long-term side effects and safety as the drug is used in larger numbers of patients with many types of diseases. Doctors can also learn more about how well the drug works and whether it might be helpful when used in other ways (such as in combination with other treatments).

What it is like to be in a clinical trial

If you participate in a clinical trial, you will have a team of cancer care experts taking care of you and watching your progress very carefully. Depending on the phase of the clinical trial, you may receive more attention (such as having more doctor visits and laboratory tests) than you would if you were treated outside of a clinical trial. Clinical trials are designed to pay close attention to you. However, there are some risks. No one involved in the study knows in advance whether the treatment will work or exactly what side effects will occur. That outcome is what the study is designed to find out. While most side effects go away in time, some may be long-lasting or even life-threatening. Keep in mind, though, that even standard treatments have side effects.

Deciding to enter a clinical trial

If you would like to take part in a clinical trial, you should begin by asking your doctor if your clinic or hospital conducts clinical trials. There are requirements you must meet to take part in any clinical trial. But whether or not you enroll in a clinical trial is completely up to you. The doctors and nurses conducting the study will explain the study to you in detail. They will go over the possible risks and benefits and give you an **informed consent** form to read and sign. The form says that you understand the clinical trial and want to take part in it. Even after you read and sign the form and after the clinical trial begins, you are free to leave the study at any time, for any reason. Taking part in a clinical trial does not keep you from getting any other medical care you may need.

To find out more about clinical trials, talk to your cancer care team. Here are some questions you might ask:

- Is there a clinical trial that I should take part in?
- What is the purpose of the study?
- How might this study benefit me?
- What is likely to happen in my case with, or without, this new treatment?
- What kinds of tests and treatments does the study involve?
- What does this treatment do? Has it been used before?
- Will I know which treatment I receive?
- What are my other choices and their pros and cons?
- How could the study affect my daily life?
- What side effects can I expect from the study? Can the side effects be controlled?
- Will I have to stay in the hospital? If so, how often and for how long?
- Will the study cost me anything? Will any of the treatment be free?
- If I am harmed as a result of the research, what treatment would I be entitled to?
- What type of long-term follow-up care is part of the study?
- Has the treatment been used to treat other types of cancer?

How can I find out more about clinical trials that might be right for me?

The American Cancer Society offers a clinical trials matching service for use by patients, their family, or friends. You can reach this service at **800-303-5691** or on the Web: **http://clinicaltrials.cancer.org**.

Based on the information you give about your cancer type, stage, and previous treatments, this service can put together a list of clinical trials that match your medical needs. The service will also ask where you live and whether you are willing to travel so that it can look for a treatment center that you can access. You can also get a list of current clinical trials by calling the National Cancer Institute's Cancer Information Service toll-free at **800-4-CANCER (800-422-6237)** or by visiting the NCI clinical trials Web site at **www.cancer .gov/clinicaltrials**.

For even more information on clinical trials, contact your American Cancer Society at **800-227-2345** or visit our Web site, **cancer.org**.

Complementary and Alternative Treatments

When you have cancer, you are likely to hear about ways to treat your cancer or relieve symptoms that are different from standard medical treatment. These treatments can include vitamins, herbs, and special diets, or acupuncture and massage— among many others. You may have a lot of questions about these treatments. Talk to your doctor about any treatment you are considering. Here are some questions to ask:

- How do I know whether the treatment is safe?
- How do I know if it works?
- Should I try one or more of these treatments?
- Will these treatments cause a problem with my standard medical treatment?
- What is the difference between complementary and alternative treatments?
- Where can I find out more about these treatments?

The terms can be confusing

Not everyone uses these terms the same way, so it can be confusing. The American Cancer Society uses **complementary medicine** to refer to medicines or treatments that are used *along with* your regular medical care. **Alternative medicine** is a treatment used *instead of* standard medical treatment.

Complementary treatments

Complementary treatment methods, for the most part, are not presented as cures for cancer. Most often they are used to help you feel better. Some methods that can be used in a complementary way are meditation to reduce stress, acupuncture to relieve pain, or peppermint tea to relieve nausea. There are many others. Some of these methods are known to help and could add to your comfort and well-being, while others have not been tested. Some have been proven not to be helpful. A few have even been found to be harmful. There are many complementary methods that you can safely use with your medical treatment to help relieve symptoms or side effects, to ease pain, and to help you enjoy life more. For example, some people find methods such as aromatherapy, massage therapy, meditation, or yoga to be useful.

Alternative treatments

Alternative treatments are methods that are used instead of standard medical care. These treatments have not been proven to be safe and effective in clinical trials. Some of these treatments may even be dangerous or have life-threatening side effects. The biggest danger in most cases is that you may lose the chance to benefit from standard treatment. Delays or interruptions in your standard medical treatment may give the cancer more time to grow.

Deciding what to do

It is easy to see why people with cancer may consider alternative treatments. You want to do all you can to fight the cancer. Sometimes, mainstream treatments such as chemotherapy can be hard to take, or they may no longer be working. Sometimes, people suggest that their treatment can cure your cancer without having serious side effects, and it is normal to want to believe them. But the truth is that most nonstandard treatments have not been tested and proven to be effective for treating cancer.

As you consider your options, here are 3 important steps you can take:

- Talk to your doctor or nurse about any treatment you are thinking about using.
- Check the list of "red flags" below.
- Contact the American Cancer Society at **800-227-2345** to learn more about complementary and alternative treatments in general and to learn more about the specific treatments you are considering.

Red flags

You can use the questions below to spot treatments or methods to avoid. A "yes" answer to any one of these questions should raise a red flag.

- Does the treatment promise a cure?
- Are you told not to use standard medical treatment?
- Is the treatment or drug a "secret" that only certain people can give?
- Does the treatment require you to travel to another country?
- Do the promoters attack the medical or scientific community?

The decision is yours

Decisions about how to treat or manage your cancer are always yours to make. If you are thinking about using a complementary or alternative method, be sure to learn about it and talk with your doctor about it. With reliable information and the support of your health care team, you may be able to safely use methods that can help you while avoiding those that could be harmful.

Treatment of Basal Cell Carcinoma

Basal cell carcinoma very rarely spreads to other parts of the body, although it can grow into nearby tissues if not treated. Several methods are used to remove or destroy these cancers. The choice may depend on factors such as the tumor size and location and the person's age, general health, and preferences.

All of the treatment methods listed here can be effective. The recurrence rates range from less than 5% for Mohs surgery to up to 10% or higher for some others, but this percentage depends on the size of the tumor. Small tumors are less likely to recur than larger ones.

Curettage and electrodesiccation

Curettage and electrodesiccation is a commonly used treatment for basal cell carcinomas smaller than 1 cm (slightly less than ½ inch) across.

Simple excision

Simple excision (cutting the tumor out) is often used to remove basal cell carcinomas, along with a **margin** of normal skin.

Mohs surgery

Mohs surgery has the best cure rate for basal cell carcinoma. It is especially useful in treating large tumors, tumors where the edges are not well defined, tumors in locations such as on or near the nose, eyes, ears, forehead, scalp, fingers, and genital area, and tumors that have come back after other treatments. However, it is also more complex and expensive than other methods.

Radiation therapy

Radiation therapy is often a good option for treating older people and for tumors on the eyelids, nose, or ears—areas that are hard to treat surgically.

Immune response modifiers, photodynamic therapy, or topical chemotherapy

These treatments are sometimes considered as options for treating superficial tumors (tumors that have not extended too deeply under the skin's surface). Close follow-up is needed because these treatments do not destroy cancer cells that are deep under the surface.

Cryosurgery

Cryosurgery can be used for some small basal cell carcinomas but is not recommended for larger tumors or those on certain parts of the nose, ears, eyelids, scalp, or legs.

Treatment of Squamous Cell Carcinoma

Most squamous cell skin cancers are found and treated at an early stage, when they can be removed or destroyed with local treatment methods. In rare cases, they may spread to lymph nodes or distant sites, in which case more intensive treatment is required.

For very small squamous cell cancers, the recurrence rate is similar to that for basal cell cancers. Larger squamous cell cancers are harder to treat, and the recurrence rates for aggressive cases of this cancer can be as high as 50%.

Simple excision

Simple excision is often used to treat squamous cell carcinomas.

Curettage and electrodesiccation

Curettage and electrodesiccation is sometimes useful in treating small squamous cell carcinomas, but it is not recommended for larger tumors.

Cryosurgery

Cryosurgery is used for some cases of squamous cell carcinoma but is not recommended for larger invasive tumors or tumors on certain parts of the nose, ears, eyelids, scalp, or legs.

Mohs surgery

Mohs surgery has the highest cure rate. It is especially useful for squamous cell carcinomas larger than 2 cm (about ⅘ inch) across or with poorly defined edges, for tumors that have come back after other treatments, for cancers that are spreading along nerves under the skin, and for cancers on certain areas of the face or genital area.

Radiation therapy

Radiation therapy is a good option for treating older adults with large cancers, especially in areas where surgery is difficult (eyelids, ears, or nose). Radiation is sometimes used after surgery (simple excision or lymph node dissection) if all of the cancer was not removed (if the surgical margins were positive) or if there is a chance that some cancer may remain. It can also be used to treat cancers that have come back after surgery and have become too large or deep to be removed surgically.

Lymph node dissection

Removing regional (nearby) lymph nodes is recommended for some squamous cell carcinomas that are large or deeply invasive and in cases where the lymph nodes feel enlarged or hard. After lymph nodes are removed, they are examined under a microscope to see whether they contain cancerous cells.

Systemic chemotherapy

Systemic chemotherapy is an option for people with squamous cell carcinoma that has spread to lymph nodes or distant organs. In some cases, it may be combined with surgery or radiation therapy.

Treatment of Actinic Keratosis

Actinic keratosis is often treated because of its potential to turn into squamous cell cancer. Because this risk is low, however, treatment is generally aimed at avoiding scars or other disfiguring marks as much as possible.

Actinic keratosis is commonly treated with cryosurgery or topical fluorouracil (5-FU). These treatments destroy the affected area of the epidermis, the outermost layer of the skin. Blood vessels and lymphatic vessels, which can serve as transports for cancer cells throughout the body, are not present in this layer, so simply destroying the affected parts of the epidermis usually cures actinic keratosis.

Other topical creams such as imiquimod or diclofenac or other localized treatments (such as shave excision, curettage and electrodesiccation, or photodynamic therapy) are also sometimes used.

Treatment of Bowen Disease

Bowen disease (squamous cell carcinoma in situ) is usually treated by simple excision. Curettage and electrodesiccation, radiation therapy, topical 5-FU, and cryosurgery are other options. Laser surgery or topical therapy may be considered in special situations.

Treatment of Merkel Cell Carcinoma

Merkel cell carcinomas are first treated with wide local excision (removal of the cancer and a wide margin of normal skin) or Mohs surgery.

Merkel cell carcinomas have a tendency to spread to lymph nodes or distant sites. Because of this tendency, even if the lymph nodes do not seem enlarged, many doctors recommend a **sentinel lymph node biopsy** to look for possible spread of cancer. For this procedure, the lymph node most likely to contain cancer if it has spread (known as the sentinel node) is removed and examined. When possible, this procedure should be done before surgery to the skin. If the sentinel node contains cancer, a full lymph node dissection (removal of all of the nearby nodes) is usually done. In either case, radiation therapy after surgery is often recommended to reduce the risk of cancer recurrence. If many lymph nodes were found to contain cancer cells, adjuvant chemotherapy may be recommended as well.

If nearby lymph nodes are enlarged at the time the cancer is diagnosed, a fine needle aspiration (FNA) biopsy may be done to determine whether they contain cancer. If cancer is found, treatment options include a lymph node dissection, radiation therapy, or a combination of the two treatments. Adjuvant treatment with chemotherapy may also be considered.

For cancers that have spread to or recur in distant sites, surgery, radiation therapy, chemotherapy, or some combination of these treatments may be used. These treatments may relieve symptoms or shrink these cancers for a time, but they rarely cure Merkel cell carcinoma that has spread beyond the skin.

Overall, the **5-year survival rate** (the percentage of people who live at least 5 years after diagnosis) for Merkel cell carcinoma is about 60%.

Your Medical Team

Your medical team comprises several people, each with a different type of expertise to contribute to your care. This list will acquaint you with the health care professionals you may encounter, depending on which treatment option and follow-up path you choose, and their areas of expertise:

Dermatologic surgeon or general surgeon

Several different types of surgeons provide treatment for skin cancer. A general surgeon is trained to operate on all parts of the body, including the skin. A dermatologic surgeon is a doctor who performs surgeries on skin cancers.

Although each type of surgeon has a different area of expertise, each plays the same role in treating people with skin cancer. If you require surgery as part of your treatment, the surgeon will perform the operation and then manage any side effects you might have. He or she will also issue a report to your other doctors to help determine the rest of your treatment plan.

Dermatologist

A dermatologist is a doctor who specializes in the diagnosis and treatment of skin problems.

Dermatopathologist

A dermatopathologist is a doctor specializing in diagnosing skin biopsies under a microscope.

Personal or primary care physician

A personal physician may be a general doctor, internist, or family practice doctor. He or she is often the medical doctor you first saw when you noticed symptoms of illness.

Plastic/reconstructive surgeon

A plastic surgeon or reconstructive surgeon is a doctor who specializes in reducing scarring or disfigurement that may occur as a result of treatment for diseases, accidents, or birth defects.

More Treatment Information

For more details on treatment options—including some that may not be addressed in this book—the National Comprehensive Cancer Network (NCCN) and the National Cancer Institute (NCI) are good sources of information.

The NCCN, made up of experts from many of the nation's leading cancer centers, develops cancer treatment guidelines for doctors to use when treating patients. Those are available on the NCCN Web site (**www.nccn.org**).

The NCI provides treatment guidelines via its telephone information center (**800-4-CANCER**) and its Web site (**www.cancer.gov**). Detailed guidelines intended for use by cancer care professionals are also available on its Web site.

Questions to Ask

What Should You Ask Your Doctor About Your Skin Cancer?

As you cope with cancer and cancer treatment, you need to have honest, open discussions with your doctor. You should feel free to ask any question that is on your mind, no matter how small it might seem. Nurses, social workers, and other members of the treatment team may also be able to answer many of your questions. Here are some questions you might want to ask:

- What type of skin cancer do I have?
- Can you explain the different types of skin cancer?
- Has my cancer spread beneath the skin? Has it spread to lymph nodes or other organs?
- Are there other tests that need to be done before we can decide on treatment?
- How much experience do you have treating this type of cancer?
- What are my treatment options? What do you recommend? Why?

- Will I be okay if the cancer is just removed with no follow-up treatment?
- What risks or side effects should I expect?
- Will I have a scar after treatment?
- What are the chances of my cancer coming back with the treatment options we have discussed? What would we do if that happens?
- What should I do to be ready for treatment?
- What is my expected prognosis, based on my cancer as you view it?
- What are my chances of another skin cancer developing?
- Should I take special precautions to avoid sun exposure? What are the most important steps I can take to protect myself from the sun?
- Are any of my family members at risk for skin cancer? What should I tell them to do? Should I tell my children's doctor that I have received a skin cancer diagnosis?

Along with these sample questions, be sure to write down your own. For instance, you might want more information about recovery times so you can plan your work schedule. Or you may want to ask about second opinions or about clinical trials for which you may qualify.

After Treatment

What Happens After Treatment for Basal and Squamous Cell Skin Cancers?

Completing treatment can be both stressful and exciting. You will be relieved to finish treatment, yet it is hard not to worry about cancer coming back. (When cancer returns, it is called recurrence.) This concern is common among those who have had cancer. It may take some time before your confidence in your own recovery begins to feel real and your fears are somewhat relieved. Even with no recurrences, people who have had cancer learn to live with uncertainty.

Follow-up Care

After your treatment is over, your doctor will likely recommend that you examine your skin once a month and protect yourself from the sun. Family members and friends can also be asked to watch for growths or suspicious areas in places that are hard for you to see.

If skin cancer does recur, it is most likely to happen in the first 5 years after treatment. In addition, a person who has had skin cancer is at higher risk for another one developing in a different location.

You should have follow-up examinations as advised by your doctor. Your schedule for follow-up visits will depend on the type of cancer you had and your specific situation. Different doctors may recommend different schedules.

- For basal cell cancers, visits are often recommended about every 6 months for the first 5 years, followed by yearly visits thereafter.
- For squamous cell cancers, visits are usually more frequent—often every 3 to 6 months for the first several years, followed by longer times between visits.

During your follow-up visits, your doctor will ask about symptoms and examine you to look for signs of recurrence or new skin cancers. For more extensive cancers, such as those that spread to lymph nodes, he or she may also order imaging tests such as CT scans or x-rays.

Follow-up is also needed to check for possible side effects of certain treatments. Ask your health care team any questions you may have and discuss any concerns at these visits. Almost any cancer treatment can have side effects. Some side effects may last for a few weeks to several months, but others can be permanent. Do not hesitate to tell your cancer care team about any symptoms or side effects that bother you so they can help you manage them.

Seeing a New Doctor

At some point after your cancer diagnosis and treatment, you may find yourself in the office of a new doctor. Your original doctor may have moved or retired, or you may have moved or changed doctors for some reason. It is important that you be able to give your new doctor the exact details of your diagnosis and treatment. Make sure you have the following information:

- a copy of pathology reports from any biopsies or surgeries
- if you had surgery, a copy of your operative report
- if you were hospitalized, a copy of the discharge summary that doctors must prepare when patients are sent home
- if you had radiation therapy, a summary of the type and dose of radiation and when and where it was given
- if you had chemotherapy, a list of your drugs, drug doses, and when you took them

It is also important to keep your health insurance. Even though no one wants to think of the cancer coming back, it is always a possibility. If it happens, the last thing you want is to have to worry about paying for treatment.

Lifestyle Changes to Consider During and After Treatment

Having cancer and dealing with treatment can be time-consuming and emotionally draining, but it can also be a time to look at your life in new ways. Maybe you are thinking about how to improve your health over the long term. Some people even begin this process during cancer treatment.

Make Healthier Choices

Think about your life before you learned you had cancer. Were there things you did that might have made you less healthy? Maybe you drank too much alcohol, or ate more than you needed, or smoked, or did not exercise very often. Emotionally, maybe you kept your feelings bottled up, or maybe you let stressful situations go on too long.

Now is not the time to feel guilty or to blame yourself. However, you can start making changes *today* that can have positive effects for the rest of your life. Not only will you feel better but you will also be healthier. What better time than now to take advantage of the motivation you have as a result of going through a life-changing experience like having cancer?

You can start by working on those things that you feel most concerned about. Get help with those that are harder for you. For instance, if you are thinking about quitting smoking and need help, call the American Cancer Society at **800-227-2345**.

Latest Research

What Is New in Research and Treatment of Basal and Squamous Cell Skin Cancers?

Research into the causes, prevention, and treatment of nonmelanoma skin cancer is under way in many medical centers throughout the world.

Basic Skin Cancer Research

Scientists have made a great deal of progress in recent years in understanding how exposure to ultraviolet (UV) radiation damages DNA and how changes in DNA cause normal skin cells to become cancerous. Researchers are continually working to apply this new information to new strategies for treating skin cancers.

Public Education

Most skin cancer is preventable. The greatest reduction in the number of skin cancer cases and in the pain and loss of life from this disease will come from preventive strategies. This means educating the public about skin cancer risk factors, prevention, and detection. It is important for health care professionals and skin cancer survivors to remind others about the dangers of excessive unprotected exposure to UV radiation (from the sun and from man-made sources such as tanning beds) and about how easily they can protect their skin from exposure to UV radiation.

The American Academy of Dermatology (AAD) sponsors annual free skin cancer screenings throughout the country. Many local American Cancer Society offices work closely with AAD to provide volunteers for registration, coordination, and education efforts related to these free screenings. Look for information in your area about these screenings or call the AAD for more information. Their phone number and Web site are listed in the "Resources" section on page 81.

Preventing Genital Skin Cancers

Squamous cell cancers that start in the genital region account for almost half of the deaths from keratinocyte cancers. Many of these cancers may be related to infection with certain types of human papilloma virus (HPV), which can be spread through sexual contact. In recent years, vaccines have been developed to help protect against infection from some types of HPV. The main intent of the vaccines has been to reduce the risk of cervical cancer, as well as the risk of other cancers that might be related to HPV, including some squamous cell cancers.

Chemoprevention

An area of active research is the field of chemoprevention, in which drugs are used to prevent cancers from forming. Chemoprevention is likely to be most useful for people at high risk for skin cancer (especially squamous cell cancers), such as those with a history of skin cancer or those who have received organ transplants.

The most widely studied drugs so far are retinoids, which are drugs related to vitamin A. They have shown some promise but can have side effects, including the potential to cause birth defects. For this reason, they are not widely used at this time, except in some people at very high risk. Further studies of retinoids are under way. Other compounds are being looked at to reduce the risk of skin cancer.

Treatment

Local treatments

Current local treatments are successful for most nonmelanoma skin cancers. Still, even some small cancers can be hard to treat if they are located in certain areas. Newer forms of non-surgical treatment such as imiquimod cream, photodynamic therapy, immune response modifiers, and laser surgery may help reduce scarring and other possible side effects of treatment. Studies are now under way to determine the best way to use these treatments and to try to improve on their effectiveness.

Treating advanced disease

Although most skin cancers are found and treated at a fairly early stage, some may spread to other parts of the body. These cancers can often be hard to treat with current therapies such as radiation and chemotherapy. Several studies are testing newer targeted drugs for advanced squamous cell cancers. Cells from these cancers often have too much of a protein called EGFR on their surfaces, which may help them grow. Drugs that target this protein, such as erlotinib (Tarceva) and gefitinib (Iressa), are now being tested in clinical trials. A drug that targets different cell proteins, known as dasatinib (Sprycel), is also being studied for advanced skin cancers.

Resources

Additional Resources
The American Cancer Society is happy to address any cancer-related topic. If you have questions, please call us at **800-227-2345**, 24 hours a day.

More Information from Your American Cancer Society
The following related information may also be helpful to you. These materials may be ordered from our toll-free number, **800-227-2345**.

Spanish language versions of some of these documents are also available.

A Parent's Guide to Skin Protection

After Diagnosis: A Guide for Patients and Families

Lasers in Cancer Treatment

Photodynamic Therapy

Skin Cancer Prevention and Early Detection

Sun Basics: Skin Protection Made Simple (information for children aged 8 to 14)

Surgery

Understanding Chemotherapy: A Guide for Patients and Their Families

Understanding Radiation Therapy: A Guide for Patients and Their Families

National Organizations and Web Sites*

In addition to the American Cancer Society, other sources of patient information and support include the following:

American Academy of Dermatology
Toll-free number: 866-503-SKIN (888-503-7546)
Internet: www.aad.org

Environmental Protection Agency
Internet: www.epa.gov/ebtpages/humasunprotection
.html

National Cancer Institute
Toll-free number: 800-422-6237 (800-4-CANCER)
TYY: 800-332-8615
Internet: www.cancer.gov

Skin Cancer Foundation
Toll-free number: 800-754-6490 (800-SKIN-490)
Internet: www.skincancer.org

References

Albert MR, Weinstock MA. Keratinocyte carcinoma. *CA Cancer J Clin.* 2003;53(5):292–302.

American Joint Committee on Cancer. Cutaneous squamous cell carcinoma and other cutaneous carcinomas. In: Edge SB, Byrd DR, Compton CC. *AJCC Cancer Staging Manual.* 7th ed. New York: Springer; 2010:301–314.

Bath-Hextall F, Bong J, Perkins W, Williams H. Interventions for basal cell carcinoma of the skin: systematic review. *BMJ.* 2004;329(7468):705–708. Epub 2004 Sept 13.

Lang PG, Maize JC. Basal cell carcinoma. In: Rigel DS, Friedman RJ, Dzubow LM, Reintgen DS, Bystryn JC, Marks R, eds. *Cancer of the Skin.* Philadelphia: Elsevier Saunders; 2005:101–132.

Inclusion on this list does not imply endorsement by the American Cancer Society.

Lewis KG, Weinstock MA. Trends in nonmelanoma skin cancer mortality rates in the United States, 1969 through 2000. *J Invest Dermatol.* 2007;127(10):2323–2327. Epub 2007 May 24.

National Cancer Institute. Physician Data Query (PDQ). Skin Cancer Treatment. 2008. National Cancer Institute Web site. www.cancer.gov/cancertopics/pdq/treatment/skin/HealthProfessional. Accessed August 3, 2009.

National Comprehensive Cancer Network (NCCN). Practice Guidelines in Oncology: Basal Cell and Squamous Cell Skin Cancers. Version 1.2009. National Comprehensive Cancer Network Web site. www.nccn.org/professionals/physician_gls/PDF/nmsc.pdf. Accessed August 3, 2009.

National Comprehensive Cancer Network (NCCN). Practice Guidelines in Oncology: Merkel Cell Carcinoma. Version 1. 2009. National Comprehensive Cancer Network Web site. www.nccn.org/professionals/physician_gls/PDF/mcc.pdf. Accessed August 3, 2009.

Nguyen TH, Yoon J. Squamous cell carcinoma. In: Rigel DS, Friedman RJ, Dzubow LM, Reintgen DS, Bystryn JC, Marks R, eds. *Cancer of the Skin.* Philadelphia: Elsevier Saunders; 2005:133–150.

Rubin AI, Chen EH, Ratner D. Basal-cell carcinoma. *N Engl J Med.* 2005;353(21):2262–2269.

Taylor G, Mollick DK, Heilman ER. Merkel cell carcinoma. In: Rigel DS, Friedman RJ, Dzubow LM, Reintgen DS, Bystryn JC, Marks R, eds. *Cancer of the Skin.* Philadelphia: Elsevier Saunders; 2005:323–327.

Thomas VD, Aasi SZ, Wilson LD, Leffell DJ. Cancer of the skin. In: DeVita VT, Lawrence TS, Rosenberg SA, eds. *DeVita, Hellman, and Rosenberg's Cancer: Principles and Practice of Oncology.* 8th ed. Philadelphia: Lippincott Williams & Wilkins; 2008:1863–1887.

Wood GS, Gunkel J, Stewart D, et al. Nonmelanoma skin cancers: basal cell and squamous cell carcinomas. In: Abeloff MD, Armitage JO, Niederhuber JE, Kastan MB, McKenna WG, eds. *Abeloff's Clinical Oncology*. 4th ed. Philadelphia: Elsevier; 2008:1253–1270.

Young JL, Ward KC, Ries LAG. Cancers of rare sites. In: Ries LAG, Young JL, Keel GE, Eisner MP, Lin YD, Horner M-J, eds. SEER Survival Monograph: Cancer Survival Among Adults: U.S. SEER Program, 1988-2001, Patient and Tumor Characteristics. National Cancer Institute, SEER Program, NIH Pub. No. 07-6215, Bethesda, MD, 2007.

Glossary

acquired immunodeficiency syndrome (AIDS): a severe immunological disorder caused by the retrovirus HIV, resulting in a defect in cell-mediated immune response that is manifested by increased susceptibility to opportunistic infections and to certain rare cancers, especially Kaposi sarcoma. It is transmitted primarily by exposure to contaminated body fluids, especially blood and semen.

actinic keratosis: a small, rough spot occurring on skin that has been chronically exposed to the sun. Actinic keratoses generally measure in size between 2 to 6 millimeters in diameter. They are usually reddish in color and often have a white scale on top. Actinic keratoses are precancerous (premalignant), and can develop into squamous cell carcinoma, although very few actually become cancerous. Also called solar keratosis.

adjuvant (AJ-uh-vunt) therapy: additional treatment given after the main treatment. It usually refers to hormone therapy, chemotherapy, radiation therapy, or immunotherapy added after surgery to increase the chances of curing the disease or to prevent it from coming back.

adnexal tumors: tumors that start in the hair follicles or glands of the skin. Malignant adnexal tumors are extremely rare, but benign adnexal tumors are common.

AJCC staging system: *see* American Joint Committee on Cancer staging system.

albinism: a rare inherited condition present at birth, characterized by a lack of pigment that normally gives color to the skin, hair, and eyes. *See also* pigment.

alternative medicine (alternative therapy): an unproven medication or therapy that is recommended instead of standard (proven) therapy. Some alternative therapies have dangerous or even life-threatening side effects. With others, the main danger is that the patient may lose the opportunity to benefit from standard therapy. The American Cancer Society recommends that patients considering the use of any alternative or complementary therapies discuss them with their cancer care team. *Compare with* complementary medicine.

American Joint Committee on Cancer (AJCC) TNM staging system: a system for describing the extent of a cancer's spread by using 0 and Roman numerals from I through IV. Also called the TNM system. *See also* staging.

anesthesia (an-es-THEE-zhuh): the loss of feeling or sensation as a result of drugs or gases. **General anesthesia** causes loss of consciousness (puts you to sleep). **Local** or **regional anesthesia** numbs only a certain area of the body. *See also* anesthetic.

anesthetic (an-es-THEH-tik): a topical or intravenous substance that causes loss of feeling or awareness in a part of the body. General anesthetics are used to put patients to sleep for procedures. *See also* anesthesia.

angiosarcoma (AN-jee-o-sar-KO-ma): a type of cancer that begins in the cells that line blood vessels or lymph vessels.

arsenic: a poisonous metallic element.

basal cell cancer: *see* basal cell carcinoma.

basal cell carcinoma: a type of skin cancer that arises from the basal cells, small round cells found in the lower part (or base) of the epidermis, the outer layer of the skin.

basal cell nevus syndrome: a genetic condition that causes unusual facial features and disorders of the skin, bones, nervous system, eyes, and endocrine glands. People with this syndrome have a higher risk of basal cell carcinoma. Also called Gorlin syndrome and nevoid basal cell carcinoma syndrome.

basal cells: small, round cells found in the lower part (or base) of the epidermis, the outer layer of the skin.

basal layer: the deepest layer of the epidermis. *See also* epidermis.

basement membrane: a very thin layer of tissue upon which is posed a single layer of cells. The basement membrane is made up of proteins held together by collagen. *See also* collagen.

benign: not cancer; not malignant.

biopsy: the removal of a sample of tissue to see whether cancer cells are present. There are several kinds of biopsies. *See also* fine needle aspiration.

> **excisional biopsy:** a surgical procedure in which an entire lump or suspicious area is removed for diagnosis. The tissue is then examined under a microscope.
> **incisional biopsy:** a surgical procedure in which a portion of a lump or suspicious area is removed for diagnosis. The tissue is then examined under a microscope.
> **punch biopsy:** removal of a small, disk-shaped sample of tissue by using a sharp, hollow device. The tissue is then examined under a microscope.
> **shave biopsy:** a procedure in which a skin abnormality and a thin layer of surrounding skin are removed with a small blade for examination under a microscope.

bone marrow: the soft, organic material in the cavities of bones, a network of blood vessels and special connective tissue fibers that hold together a composite of fat and blood-producing cells.

Bowen disease: *see* squamous cell carcinomas in situ.

cancer: cancer is not just one disease but a group of diseases. All forms of cancer cause cells in the body to change and grow out of control. Most types of cancer cells form a lump or mass called a tumor. The tumor can invade and destroy healthy tissue. Cells from the tumor can break away and travel to other parts of the body, where they can continue to grow. This spreading process is called metastasis. When cancer spreads, it is still named after the part of the body where it started. For example, if breast cancer spreads to the lungs, it is still called breast cancer, not lung cancer.

Some cancers, such as blood cancers, do not form a tumor. Not all tumors are cancer. A tumor that is not cancer is called benign. Benign tumors do not grow and spread the way cancer does. Benign tumors are usually not a threat to life. Another word for cancerous is malignant.

cancer care team: the group of health care professionals who work together to identify, treat, and care for people with cancer. The cancer care team may include the following and others: primary care physicians, pathologists, oncology specialists (medical oncologist, radiation oncologist), surgeons, nurses, oncology nurse specialists, and oncology social workers. Whether the team is linked formally or informally, there is usually one person who takes the job of coordinating the team.

cancer cell: a cell that divides and reproduces abnormally and has the potential to spread throughout the body, crowding out normal cells and tissue. *See also* metastasis, cancer.

carcinoma: any cancerous tumor that begins in the lining layer of organs. At least 80% of all cancers are carcinomas.

cell: the basic unit of which all living things are made. Cells replace themselves by splitting and forming new cells (mitosis). The processes that control the formation of new cells and the death of old cells are disrupted in cancer.

chemotherapy (key-mo-THAYR-uh-pee): treatment with drugs to destroy cancer cells. Chemotherapy is often used, either alone or with surgery or radiation, to treat cancer that has spread or recurred, or when there is a strong chance that it could recur. **Systemic chemotherapy** refers to treatment that reaches and affects cells throughout the entire body. **Topical chemotherapy** refers to treatment with anticancer drugs in a lotion or cream applied to the skin.

clinical trials: research studies to test new drugs or treatments to compare current, standard treatments with others that may be better. Before a new treatment is used on people, it is studied in the laboratory. If laboratory studies suggest the treatment will work, the next step is to test its value for patients. These human studies are called clinical trials. *See also* control group.

collagen: a fibrous protein that is the major constituent of cartilage and other connective tissue.

complementary medicine (complementary therapy): treatment used in addition to standard therapy. Some complementary therapies may help relieve certain symptoms of cancer, relieve side effects of standard cancer therapy, or improve a person's sense of well-being. The American Cancer Society recommends that patients considering the use of any alternative or complementary therapies discuss these therapies with their cancer care team, since many of these treatments are unproven and some can be harmful. *Compare with* alternative medicine.

computed tomography (to-MAHG-ruh-fee): an imaging test in which many x-rays are taken of a part of the body from different angles. These images are combined by a computer to produce cross-sectional pictures of internal organs. Except for the injection of a contrast dye (needed in some but not all cases), this is a painless procedure that can be done in an outpatient clinic. It is often referred to as a "CT" or "CAT" scan.

congenital: present at and existing from the time of birth.

control group: in research or clinical trials, the group that does not receive the treatment being tested. The group may get a placebo or sham treatment, or it may receive standard therapy. Also called the comparison group. *See also* clinical trials.

cryosurgery: a procedure involving the use of subfreezing temperatures to destroy tissue. Also called cryotherapy.

CT scan or CAT scan: *see* computed tomography.

curettage and electrodessication: the removal of tissue or growths by scraping with a curette to improve examination or for removal. A needle-shaped electrode is then used to treat the area with an electric current that stops the bleeding and destroys cancer cells that remain around the edge of the wound. The process may be repeated one to three times during the surgery to remove all of the cancer. *See also* curette.

curette: a surgical instrument shaped like a scoop or spoon, used to remove tissue or growths from a body cavity. *See also* curettage and electrodessication.

cutaneous T-cell lymphoma: a rare cancer of the white blood cells that primarily affects the skin and only secondarily affects other sites. *See also* lymphoma.

dermatofibrosarcoma protuberans (DFSP): a slow-growing abnormal formation of skin tissue consisting of one or more purplish nodules that tends to recur but usually does not metastasize.

dermatoscopy: an examination technique that uses a hand-held skin surface microscope. The skin surface is illuminated by a halogen bulb and the glass disc of the scope is pressed against the skin, making details of the epidermis visible. Also known as dermatoscopy. *See also* epiluminescence microscopy (ELM).

dermis: the lower or inner layer of the two main layers of tissue that make up the skin.

diagnosis: identifying a disease by its signs or symptoms and by using imaging procedures and laboratory findings. For some types of cancer, the earlier a diagnosis is made, the better the chance for long-term survival.

dihydroxyacetone (DHA): the active chemical ingredient in sunless tanning lotions. When applied to the skin, DHA reacts with the amino acids in the skin and causes the pigment to darken.

DNA: deoxyribonucleic acid. DNA is the genetic "blueprint" found in the nucleus of each cell. It holds genetic information on cell growth, division, and function.

epidermis: the upper or outer layer of the two main layers of tissue that make up the skin.

epiluminescence microscopy (ELM): a technique that uses a hand-held magnifying lens to examine the skin and determine whether cancer is present in pigmented skin lesions. *See also* dermatoscopy.

excisional biopsy: *see* biopsy.

external beam radiation therapy (EBRT): radiation that is focused from a source outside the body on the area affected by the cancer. It is much like getting a diagnostic x-ray, but for a longer period.

FDA: *see* U.S. Food and Drug Administration.

fibroblasts: connective tissue cells that make and secrete collagen proteins. *See also* collagen.

fine needle aspiration: a procedure in which a thin needle is used to draw up (aspirate) samples for examination under a microscope. *See also* biopsy.

5-fluorouracil: a drug in a cream form that is used to treat certain skin conditions by stopping cells from making DNA. This drug may also kill cancer cells. Also called 5-FU and fluorouracil.

five (5)-year survival rate: the percentage of people with a given cancer who are expected to survive 5 years or longer with the disease. Five-year survival rates have some drawbacks. Although the rates are based on the most recent information available, they may include data from patients treated several years earlier. Advances in cancer treatment often occur quickly. Five-year survival rates, while statistically valid, may not reflect these advances. They should not be seen as a predictor in an individual case.

genes: segments of DNA that contains information on hereditary characteristics such as hair color, eye color, and height, as well as susceptibility to certain diseases. *See also* DNA.

hemangioma: abnormal buildup of blood vessels in the skin or internal organs.

human immunodeficiency virus (HIV): a type of retrovirus that causes acquired immunodeficiency syndrome (AIDS). It is transmitted through contact with an infected individual's blood, semen, cervical secretions, cerebrospinal fluid, or synovial fluid. The virus infects T-helper cells of the immune system and results in infection with a long incubation period, averaging 10 years. *See also* acquired immunodeficiency syndrome (AIDS).

human papilloma virus: a member of a family of viruses that can cause abnormal tissue growth (for example, genital warts) and other changes to cells. Infection with certain types of human papillomavirus increases the risk of developing cervical cancer. Also called HPV.

immune response modifier: a manufactured substance, such as imiquimod, that is designed to strengthen, direct, or restore the body's immune response against infection or cancer.

immunotherapy: treatment to boost or restore the ability of the immune system to fight cancer, infections, and other diseases. Also used to lessen certain side effects that may be caused by some cancer treatments. Agents used in immunotherapy include monoclonal antibodies, growth factors, and vaccines. These agents may also have a direct antitumor effect. Also called biological response modifier therapy, biological therapy, biotherapy, and BRM therapy.

incisional biopsy: *see* biopsy.

informed consent: a legal document that explains a course of treatment, the risks, benefits, and possible alternatives; the process by which patients agree to treatment.

in situ (in SIGH-too): in place; localized and confined to one area. A very early stage of cancer.

interferon: a type of immunotherapy that uses a synthetic protein that resembles a protein that occurs naturally in the body. Interferon is given as an injection just under the skin, usually in the thigh or abdomen. Interferon is given to slow down or stop cancer cells dividing, to reduce the ability of cancer cells to protect themselves from the immune system, and to strengthen the body's immune system. *See also* immunotherapy.

Kaposi sarcoma: a type of cancer characterized by the abnormal growth of blood vessels that develop into skin lesions or occur internally.

keratin: a tough, insoluble protein found in the outer layer of the skin.

keratinoctye cancer: *see* keratinocyte carcinoma.

keratinocyte carcinoma: cancer that starts in an epidermal cell that produces keratin. Basal cell carcinoma and squamous cell carcinoma are the most common types of keratinocyte carcinomas.

keratinocytes: cells found in the outer layer of the skin that produce keratin, a tough insoluble protein.

keratoacanthoma (KAYR-uh-toh-AK-un-THO-muh): a rapidly growing, dome-shaped skin tumor that usually occurs on sun-exposed areas of the body, especially around the head and neck. Keratoacanthoma occurs more often in males. Although in most people it goes away on its own, in a few people it comes back. Rarely, it may spread to other parts of the body.

laser surgery: a surgical procedure that uses the cutting power of a laser beam to make bloodless cuts in tissue or to remove a surface lesion such as a tumor.

lipoma: a benign tumor made of fat cells.

lymphedema: swelling due to a collection of excess fluid in the arms or legs. This may happen after the lymph nodes and vessels are removed or are injured by radiation, or it can happen many years after treatment. It may also happen when a tumor disrupts normal fluid drainage. Lymphedema can persist and interfere with activities of daily living. *See also* lymph nodes.

lymph nodes: small, bean-shaped collections of immune system tissue that are found along lymphatic vessels. They remove cell waste, germs, and other harmful substances from lymph. They help fight infections and also have a role in fighting cancer, although cancers sometimes spread through lymph nodes. Also called lymph glands.

lymphocyte: a type of white blood cell that helps the body fight infection.

lymphoma: a cancer of the lymphatic system, a network of thin vessels and nodes throughout the body. Its function is to fight infection. Lymphoma involves a type of white blood cells called lymphocytes. The 2 main types of lymphoma are Hodgkin disease and non-Hodgkin lymphoma. The treatment methods for these 2 types of lymphomas are very different. *See also* lymphocyte.

magnetic resonance imaging (MRI): a method of taking pictures of the inside of the body. Instead of using x-rays, MRI uses a powerful magnet to send radio waves through the body. The images appear on a computer screen, as well as on film. Like x-rays, the procedure is physically painless, but some people may feel confined inside the MRI machine, and it is noisy.

malignant: cancerous.

malignant tumor: a mass of cancer cells that may invade surrounding tissues or spread (metastasize) to distant sites in the body. *See also* tumor, metastasis, metastatic cancer.

margin: the edge of the cancerous tissue removed during surgery. A negative surgical margin is a sign that no cancer was left behind. A positive surgical margin means that cancer cells are found at the outer edge of the removed sample and is usually a sign some cancer is still in the body.

melanin: a pigment that gives color to skin and eyes and helps protect them from damage by ultraviolet rays.

melanocytes: cells in the skin and eyes that produce and contain the pigment called melanin.

melanoma: a form of cancer that begins in melanocytes. It may begin in a mole (skin melanoma), but can also begin in other pigmented tissues, such as in the eye or in the intestines.

Merkel cell carcinoma: a rare type of skin cancer that usually appears as a flesh-colored or bluish-red nodule, often on the face, head, or neck. Merkel cell carcinoma tends to grow fast and to spread quickly to other parts of the body. Merkel cell carcinoma is named after the Merkel cell, which is found at the base of the outermost layer of your skin (epidermis). *See also* Merkel cell polyomavirus.

Merkel cell polyomavirus (MCV): the virus that is suspected to cause most cases of Merkel cell carcinoma.

metastasis: cancer cells that have spread to one or more sites elsewhere in the body, often by way of the lymphatic system or bloodstream. **Regional metastasis** is cancer that has spread to the lymph nodes, tissues, or organs close to the primary site. **Distant metastasis** is cancer that has spread to organs or tissues that are farther away (such as when skin cancer spreads to the lungs). The plural of this word is metastases. *See also* lymph nodes, metastasize, metastatic.

metastasize: the spread of cancer cells to one or more sites elsewhere in the body, often by way of the lymphatic system or bloodstream. *See also* metastasis.

metastatic cancer: a way to describe cancer that has spread from the primary site (where it started) to other structures or organs, nearby or far away. *See also* metastasis, metastasize.

Mohs surgery: a surgical procedure used to treat skin cancer. Individual layers of cancerous tissue are removed and examined under a microscope one at a time until all cancerous tissue has been removed. Also called Mohs micrographic surgery.

mole: a benign (noncancerous) growth on the skin that is formed by a cluster of melanocytes (cells that make a substance called melanin, which gives color to skin and eyes). A mole is usually dark and may be raised from the skin. Also called nevus.

MRI: *see* magnetic resonance imaging.

mycosis fungoides (my-KOH-sis fun-GOY-deez): a type of non-Hodgkin lymphoma that first appears on the skin and can spread to the lymph nodes or other organs such as the spleen, liver, or lungs.

neuroendocrine cells: cells that release hormones into the blood in response to stimulation of the nervous system.

nonmelanoma skin cancer: skin cancer that forms in basal cells or squamous cells but not in melanocytes (pigment-producing cells of the skin).

nonsteroidal anti-inflammatory drug: a drug that decreases fever, swelling, pain, and redness. Also called NSAID.

papillomas: benign growths on the skin or mucous membrane. Viruses that cause these growths are called human papillomaviruses (HPVs).

photodynamic therapy (PDT): treatment with drugs that become active when exposed to light. These activated drugs may kill cancer cells.

pigment: a substance that gives color to tissue. Pigments are responsible for the color of skin, eyes, and hair.

primary cutaneous lymphoma: a type of lymphoma that starts in the skin. Cutaneous T-cell lymphoma is the most common type of primary cutaneous lymphoma. *See also* mycosis fungoides.

prognosis: a prediction of the course of disease; the outlook for the chances of survival.

psoriasis: a chronic disease of the immune system that appears on the skin marked by red patches covered with white scales. Psoriasis is not malignant or contagious but is associated with other serious health conditions such as diabetes and heart disease.

punch biopsy: *see* biopsy.

radiation therapy: treatment with high-energy rays (such as x-rays) to kill or shrink cancer cells. The radiation may come from outside of the body (external radiation) or from radioactive materials placed directly in the tumor (brachytherapy or internal radiation). Radiation therapy may be used as the main treatment for a cancer, to reduce the size of a cancer before surgery, or to destroy any remaining cancer cells after surgery. In advanced cancer cases, it may also be used as palliative treatment.

recurrence: the return of cancer after treatment. **Local recurrence** means that the cancer has come back at the same place as the original cancer. **Regional recurrence** means that the cancer has come back after treatment in the lymph nodes near the primary site. **Distant recurrence**, also known as metastatic recurrence, is when cancer metastasizes after treatment to distant organs or tissues (such as the lungs, liver, bone marrow, or brain). *See also* metastasis, metastasize, metastatic.

regional metastasis: *see* metastasis.

risk factor: anything that affects a person's chance of getting a disease such as cancer. Different cancers have different risk factors. For example, unprotected exposure to strong sunlight is a risk factor for skin cancer; smoking is a risk factor for lung, mouth, larynx, and other cancers. Some risk factors, such as smoking, can be controlled. Others, like a person's age, cannot be changed.

sarcomas: cancers of the bone, cartilage, fat, muscle, blood vessels, or other connective or supportive tissue.

seborrheic keratoses: benign raised growths on the skin, usually brown, black, or pale and often appearing on the face, chest, shoulders, or back. The growth has a waxy, scaly, slightly elevated appearance. Occasionally, a single growth appears, but multiple growths are more common. Typically, seborrheic keratoses don't become cancerous, but they can look like skin cancer. Seborrheic keratoses are common noncancerous (benign) skin growths in older adults.

sentinel lymph node biopsy: a diagnostic procedure involving the removal of the first lymph node to which cancer cells are likely to spread from the primary tumor. In some cases, there can be more than one sentinel lymph node. For this procedure, a radioactive substance or contrast dye is injected near the tumor. A scanner is then used to map the circulation of the substance through the sentinel node. The node is then removed and examined for the presence of cancer cells. *See also* lymph node.

shave biopsy: *see* biopsy.

sign: an observable physical change caused by an illness. *Compare with* symptom.

simple excision: a surgical procedure in which a local anesthetic is used to remove a skin lesion.

skin biopsy: *see* biopsy.

solar keratosis: *see* actinic keratosis.

squamous cell cancer: *see* squamous cell carcinoma.

squamous cell carcinoma: cancer that begins in squamous cells, which are thin, flat cells that look like fish scales. Squamous cells are found in the tissue that forms the surface of the skin, the lining of the hollow organs of the body, and the passages of the respiratory and digestive tracts.

squamous cell carcinoma in situ: cancer that begins in squamous cells and is confined to the site of origin and has neither invaded neighboring tissues nor metastasized to other sites. A very early stage of skin cancer. Also called Bowen disease. *See also* squamous cell carcinoma.

squamous cells: flat cells that looks like a fish scale under a microscope. These cells are found in the tissues that form the surface of the skin, the lining of the hollow organs of the body (such as the bladder, kidney, and uterus), and the passages of the respiratory and digestive tracts.

stage: the extent of a cancer in the body. *See* staging.

staging: the process of finding out whether cancer has spread and, if so, how far. The TNM system, which is used most often, gives 3 key pieces of information:

- T refers to the size of the tumor
- N describes how far the cancer has spread to nearby lymph nodes
- M shows whether the cancer has spread (metastasized) to other organs of the body

Letters or numbers after the T, N, and M give more details about each of these factors. To make this information more clear, the TNM descriptions can be grouped together into a simpler set of stages, labeled with Roman numerals (usually from I to IV). In general, the lower the number, the less the cancer has spread. A higher number means a more serious cancer. *See also* American Joint Committee on Cancer (AJCC) TNM staging system.

stratum corneum: the outermost layer of the epidermis, which is made up of dead, flat skin cells. The stratum corneum serves as an important barrier, keeping molecules from passing into and out of the skin and thus protecting the lower layers of the skin.

subcutis: the deeper layer of the dermis, containing mostly fat and connective tissue.

sun protection factor (SPF): a number on a scale for rating sunscreens. The SPF rating is calculated by comparing the amount of time needed to produce a sunburn on protected skin to the amount of time needed to cause a sunburn on unprotected skin. Sunscreens with an SPF of 15 or higher are generally thought to provide useful protection from the sun's harmful rays.

surgical margin: *see* margin.

symptom: a change in the body caused by an illness, as described by the person experiencing it. *Compare with* sign.

systemic chemotherapy: *see* chemotherapy.

tissue: a collection of cells, united to perform a particular function in the body.

TNM staging system: *see* staging.

topical chemotherapy: *see* chemotherapy.

tumor: an abnormal lump or mass of tissue. Tumors can be benign (noncancerous) or malignant (cancerous).

tumor suppressor genes: genes that slow down cell division or cause cells to die at the appropriate time. Alterations of these genes can lead to too much cell growth and development of cancer.

ultraviolet protection factor (UPF): a number on a scale for rating sun-protective clothing for its ability to protect against ultraviolet radiation. The level of protection the garment provides from the sun's UV radiation is rated on a scale from 15 to 50+. The higher the UPF, the higher the protection from UV radiation.

ultraviolet radiation: invisible rays that are part of the energy that comes from the sun. Ultraviolet radiation also comes from sun lamps and tanning beds. It can damage the skin and cause melanoma and other types of skin cancer. Also called UV radiation.

U.S. Food and Drug Administration (FDA): an agency of the United States Department of Health and Human Services. The FDA is responsible for regulating drugs, tobacco products, biological medical products, blood products, medical devices, and radiation-emitting devices, along with other products.

UV Index: a scale ranging from 0 through 11+, used in estimating the risk for sunburn that an unprotected fair-skinned person would have if exposed to the ultraviolet radiation in midday sunlight, accounting for conditions such as cloud cover, ozone, and location.

vitamin D: a nutrient that the body needs in small amounts to function and stay healthy. Vitamin D helps the body use calcium and phosphorus to make strong bones and teeth. It is fat-soluble (can dissolve in fats and oils) and is found in fatty fish, egg yolks, and dairy products. Skin exposed to sunshine can also make vitamin D. Not enough vitamin D can cause a bone disease called rickets. It is being studied in the prevention and treatment of some types of cancer. Also called cholecalciferol.

warts: raised growths on the surface of the skin or other organ.

xeroderma pigmentosum (XP): a genetic condition marked by an extreme sensitivity to ultraviolet radiation, including sunlight. People with xeroderma pigmentosum are not able to repair skin damage from the sun and other sources of ultraviolet radiation and have a very high risk of skin cancer.

x-ray: one form of radiation that can be used at low levels to produce an image of the body on film or at high levels to destroy cancer cells.

Index

A

acquired immunodeficiency syndrome, 9
actinic keratoses
  definition of, 11
  reducing risk for, 26
  as source for squamous cell carcinoma, 7
  treatment for, 43, 46, 47, 48, 66–67
adnexal tumors, 8, 10, 34
age, 17, 18
albinism, 17
alternative therapy, 59–62
American Academy of Dermatology, 78
American Cancer Society, as resource for information about
  chemotherapy, 51
  clinical trials, 59
  complementary and alternative therapies, 62
  Kaposi sarcoma, 9
  lymphedema, 45
  lymphoma of the skin, 10
  radiation therapy, 50
  skin cancer detection, 29, 30
  skin cancer prevention, 29, 30
  smoking cessation, 76
American Joint Committee on Cancer TNM system, 39–41

angiosarcoma, 10
arsenic, 18, 29

B

babies, protecting, from sun exposure, 28
basal cell carcinoma, description of, 6–7
basal cell nevus syndrome, 19, 50
basal cells, 4
basement membrane, 5
benign skin tumors, 2, 3, 12
biopsy, lymph node, 37–38, 67–68
biopsy, skin, 36–37
bleeding of skin cancers, 33
Bowen disease, 11–12, 67

C

cancer. *See also specific names of cancers*
  definition of, 1
  DNA in, 2
  inherited, 2
cancer, skin, understanding, 3–13. *See also specific names of cancers*
cancer care team, 39, 51, 52, 55, 68–69
causes of skin cancers, 20–22
cells, types of
  abnormal, 1, 21–22
  basal cells, 4

cancer, 1, 2
  damaged, 21
  fibroblasts, 5
  keratinocytes, 4
  lymphocytes, 9–10
  melanocytes, 5, 6
  neuroendocrine cells, 8
  normal, 1
  squamous cells, 4
cetuximab, 80
check-up, skin, 30–31
chemicals, harmful, avoiding,
    18, 29
chemoprevention, 78–79
chemotherapy
  systemic, 50–51, 66
  topical, 47, 64
children
  protecting, from sun
      exposure, 28
  who have undergone
      previous radiation
      therapy, 18
classification of disease,
    39–41
clinical trials, 52–59
  deciding about, 57–58
  focus of, 52–53
  matching service, 59
  participation in, 57
  phases of, 53–56
  purpose of, 52
  questions to ask about, 58
  risks of, 57
clothing, as protection against
    radiation, 23–24
complementary therapies,
    59–62

corticosteroid drugs, 20
cryosurgery (cryotherapy),
    46, 64, 65, 66, 67
curettage and electrodesic-
    cation, 44, 63, 65, 67
cutaneous lymphoma, 8,
    9–10, 15
cutaneous T-cell lymphoma,
    10

D

dasatinib, 80
death, 13, 78
dermatofibrosarcoma
    protuberans, 10
dermatologist, 28, 35,
    36, 69
dermatopathologist, 69
dermatoscopy, 35–36
dermis, 5
dermoscopy, 35–36
detection, 30–31
diagnosis, 33–38
  biopsy, lymph node,
      37–38
  biopsy, skin, 36–37
  medical history, 35–36
  physical examination,
      35–36
  signs and symptoms, 31,
      33–34
diclofenac, 47, 67
dihydroxyacetone, 26
DNA, damage to, 2, 16,
    21–22
drugs
  clinical trials of, 52–59
  research on, 79–80

E

EGFR (epidermal growth factor receptor), 80
epidermis, 4
epiluminescence microscopy, 35–36
examination
  physical, 35
  post-treatment, 73–74
excision, shave, 44
excision, simple, 43–44, 63, 65, 67
excisional biopsy, 37, 38
exposures as risk factors. *See also* risk factors for basal and squamous cell cancer
  chemical, 18
  radiation therapy, 18
  ultraviolet radiation, 15, 16–17, 20–21, 72

F

fine needle aspiration biopsy, 37–38, 68
5-fluorouracil, 47
follow-up care, 64, 73–74

G

gefitinib, 80
gender as risk factor, 18
genes
  mutated, 2, 16, 21–22
  tumor suppressor, 21–22
genital skin cancers and precancerous lesions, 7, 12, 20, 34

preventing, 78
treatment for, 63, 65
grafting, skin, 45

H

hats as protection against radiation, 24–25, 28
health care providers, 39, 51, 52, 55, 68–69
healthier choices, making, 75
hemangiomas, 12
high-risk features in staging, 40
human immunodeficiency virus (HIV), 9, 38
human papilloma virus (HPV) infection, 20, 22, 78

I

imaging, diagnostic, 38–39, 74
imiquimod, 48, 67, 79
immune response modifier, 48, 64, 79
immunity, reduced, as risk factor, 9, 13, 19–20, 38
immunotherapy, 48, 64
incidence, 12–13
incisional biopsy, 37
interferon, 48

K

Kaposi sarcoma, 9, 34
keratinocytes, 4
keratoses, seborrheic, 12. *See also* actinic keratoses

L

laser surgery, 48, 67, 79
lifestyle changes during and after treatment, 75–76

lip balm, 25
lipomas, 12
lymphedema, 45
lymph node
    biopsy of, 37–38, 67–68
    dissection of, 66
    surgery on, 45
lymphoma, cutaneous, 8,
        9–10, 15. *See also*
        mycosis fungoides

M

medical history in diagnosis,
        35–36
medical team, 39, 51, 52, 55,
        68–69
melanocytes, 5, 6
melanoma, 5–6
Merkel cell carcinoma, 8–9
    appearance, 34
    staging of, 39
    survival rate, 68
    therapy for, 43, 45, 49, 50,
        67–68
Merkel cell polyomavirus, 8–9
metastasis
    classification of, 39, 41
    definition of, 2
    therapy for, 50–51, 68
microscopy, epiluminescence
        or surface, 35–36
Mohs surgery, 44, 63, 65
moles, 6, 12, 30, 31, 35
mortality, 13, 78
mycosis fungoides, 10, 34

N

National Cancer Institute,
        69–70

National Comprehensive
        Cancer Network, 69–70
nausea and vomiting, 51
nodes, lymph, 6, 9–10, 35.
        See also biopsy, lymph
        node; sentinel lymph
        node biopsy
nodes, lymph, classification
        of, 39–41
nonsteroidal anti-
        inflammatory drug
        (NSAID), 47
non-surgical treatments,
        developments in, 79–80

O

outdoor exposure, hours
        to avoid, 27. *See also*
        radiation, ultraviolet,
        exposure; SPF (sun
        protection factor);
        sunscreen

P

pain of skin cancers, 33
p53 gene, 21–22
photodynamic therapy, 46,
        64, 67, 79
physical examination in
        diagnosis, 35–36
physician, primary care or
        personal, 69
physicians on medical team,
        68–69
post-treatment care, 73–76.
        See also recurrence
    considering lifestyle changes
        during, 75–76
    follow-up care, 73–74

making healthier choices during, 76
seeing a new doctor, 75
precancerous skin conditions, 10–12
actinic keratosis, 11
Bowen disease, 11–12, 67
squamous cell carcinoma in situ, 11–12, 67
prevention, 23–30. *See also* chemoprevention; children, protecting, from sun exposure; ultraviolet radiation, protecting against
chemicals, harmful, avoiding, 29
chemoprevention, 78–79
in children, 28
of genital skin cancers, 78
learning more about, 29–30
research, 77–79
sunscreen for, 25–26
tanning, commercial, avoiding, 28
ultraviolet radiation, limiting exposure to, 23–29
vitamin D, 28–29
primary cutaneous lymphoma, 10
prognosis, asking physician about, 72
psoriasis treatment, as risk factor, 19
PTCH gene, 22
public education research, 77–78
punch biopsy, 36

Q
questions to ask physician, 71–72

R
radiation, ultraviolet, exposure, 15, 16–17, 20–21, 72
radiation therapy, 48–50, 65–66
radiation therapy, as risk factor, 18
reconstructive surgery, 45
recurrence, 73–74
defined, 73
and radiation therapy, 49
after treatment for basal cell carcinoma, 63
after treatment for Merkel cell carcinoma, 67
after treatment for squamous cell carcinoma, 64
research, 77–80
on chemoprevention, 78–79
clinical trials, 52–59
on DNA damage, 21, 77
on key prevention/detection strategies, 77–78
on preventing genital skin cancers, 78
on treatment, 79–80
on vitamin D, 29
retinoids, 79
risk factors for basal and squamous cell cancer, 15–22
age, 17, 18

basal cell nevus syndrome, 19, 50
fair skin, 17
gender, male, 18
human papilloma virus infection, 20, 22, 78
immunity, reduced, 19–20
inflammation, severe skin, 18–19
injury, skin, 18–19
psoriasis treatment, 19
radiation therapy exposure, 18, 49–50
sex, male, 18
skin cancer, previous, 18, 49–50, 74
smoking, 20
sunburns, 21
ultraviolet radiation exposure, 15, 16–17, 20–21
xeroderma pigmentosum, 19, 22

S

sarcomas, 8, 10, 34
screening, 30, 78
seborrheic keratosis, 12
self-examinations, skin, 30–31, 73
sentinel lymph node biopsy, 67
shade, seeking, 27
shave biopsy, 36
shave excision, 44
side effects
   of alternative therapy, 61
   checking for posttreatment, 74
   in clinical trials, 53, 55, 56, 57, 58
   of chemotherapy, 47, 51
   of radiation, 49–50
   of retinoids, 79
signs and symptoms
   of actinic keratosis, 11
   of basal cell carcinoma, 31, 33–34
   of recurrence, 74
   of Merkel cell carcinoma, 8–9
   of other skin cancers, 34
   of squamous cell carcinoma, 31, 33–34
simple excision, 43–44, 63, 65, 67
skin, fair, as risk factor, 17
skin, normal, 3–5
skin cancer, previous, as risk factor, 18, 49–50, 74
skin cancer, types of, overview, 5–12
skin examination, 30–31, 73
skin grafting, 45
smoking, 2, 20, 76
solar keratosis. *See* actinic keratoses
SPF (sun protection factor), 25–26
squamous cell carcinoma, description of, 7–8
squamous cell carcinoma in situ, 11–12
squamous cells, 4
stage grouping, 41
staging, 38–41

American Joint Committee on Cancer TNM system, 39–41

definition of, 38

physical examination as part of, 39

statistics about skin cancers, 12–13

stratum corneum, 4

subcutis, 5

sunburns, 21. *See also* ultraviolet radiation; ultraviolet radiation, protecting against

sunglasses, 26

sunlight, 16, 27. *See also* ultraviolet radiation; ultraviolet radiation, protecting against

sun protection factor (SPF), 25

sunscreen, 25–26

sun sensitivity from drug treatment, 47

surface microscopy, 35

surgeon, 68, 69

surgery

cryosurgery, 46, 64, 65, 66, 67

curettage and electrodesiccation, 44, 63, 65, 67

excision, shave, 44

excision, simple, 43–44, 63, 65, 67

lymph node, 45

Mohs, 44, 63, 65

reconstructive, 45

skin grafting, 45

survival rate, five-year, 68

swimsuits, sun-protective, for children, 28

symptoms. *See* signs and symptoms

T

tanning, commercial, 16, 21, 28

tanning beds, booths, or lamps, 16, 21, 28

tanning lotions, sunless, 26

team, medical, 68–69

treatment, adjuvant, 49

treatment. *See also* post-treatment; treatment, types of; treatment description

questions to ask physician about, 71–72

research about, 79–80

risk of recurrence with, 63, 64

side effects of, 50–51

treatment, types of, 43–68. *See also* post-treatment; treatment description; *see also* names of specific diseases

alternative, 59–62

chemotherapy, systemic, 50–51, 66

chemotherapy, topical, 47, 64

clinical trials, 52–59

complementary, 59–62

cryosurgery (cryotherapy), 46, 64, 65, 66, 67

curettage and electrodes-
iccation, 44, 63, 65, 67
excision, simple, 43–44, 63,
65, 67
immunotherapy, 48, 64
laser surgery, 48, 67, 79
lymph node dissection, 66
Mohs surgery, 44, 63, 65
non-surgical, developments
in, 79–80
other therapy, 46
photodynamic therapy, 46,
64, 67, 79
radiation therapy, 48–50,
65–66
surgery, 43–45, 48, 63,
65, 67
treatment description
for actinic keratosis, 46, 48,
66–67
for basal cell carcinoma,
63–64
for Bowen disease, 67
for Merkel cell carcinoma,
49, 67–68
for squamous cell cancers,
64–66
tumors. *See also* treatment,
types of; treatment
description; *specific
names of tumors; specific
names of treatments*
benign, 3, 12
classification of, 39–41
formation of, 2
tumor suppressor genes,
21–22

U
ultraviolet protection factor
(UPF), 24
ultraviolet radiation, 15,
16–17, 20–21, 72
clothing as protection
against, 23–24
limiting exposure to, 23–27
protecting babies and
children from, 28
ultraviolet radiation,
protecting against
advice from the American
Cancer Society on, 29
with clothing, 23–24
exposure in children, 28
with hats, 24–25
with sunglasses, 26
with sunscreen, 25–26
UPF (ultraviolet protection
factor), 24
U.S. Food and Drug
Administration
sunscreen labeling rules of,
25–26
UV (ultraviolet) index, 27
UV (ultraviolet) rays. *See*
ultraviolet radiation;
ultraviolet radiation,
protecting against

V
vitamin D, 28–29

W
warts, 12, 20
Web sites, 82

for American Academy of
Dermatology (www.aad
.org), 78, 82
for UV (ultraviolet) index
(www.epa.gov/sunwise/
uvindex.html), 27
for cancer information
(www.cancer.org), 9

for treament options
(www.nccn.org and
www.cancer.gov), 70

X

xeroderma pigmentosum,
19, 22

Books Published
by the American Cancer Society

Available everywhere books are sold and online at
www.cancer.org/bookstore

Information

The American Cancer Society: A History of Saving Lives

American Cancer Society's Complete Guide to Colorectal Cancer

American Cancer Society Complete Guide to Complementary & Alternative Cancer Therapies, Second Edition

American Cancer Society Complete Guide to Nutrition for Cancer Survivors: Eating Well, Staying Well During and After Cancer, Second Edition

American Cancer Society's Complete Guide to Prostate Cancer

Breast Cancer Clear & Simple: All Your Questions Answered

The Cancer Atlas (available in English, Spanish, French, and Chinese)

Cancer: What Causes It, What Doesn't

QuickFACTS™ —Advanced Cancer

QuickFACTS™ —Bone Metastasis

QuickFACTS™ —Colorectal Cancer, Second Edition

QuickFACTS™ —Lung Cancer

QuickFACTS™ —Melanoma

QuickFACTS™ —Prostate Cancer, Second Edition

QuickFACTS™ —Thyroid Cancer

The Tobacco Atlas, Second Edition (available in English, Spanish and French)

Day-to-Day Help

American Cancer Society Complete Guide to Family Caregiving, Second Edition

American Cancer Society's Guide to Pain Control: Understanding and Managing Cancer Pain, Revised Edition

Cancer Caregiving A to Z: An At-Home Guide for Patients and Families

Caregiving: A Step-By-Step Resource for Caring for the Person with Cancer at Home, Revised Edition

Get Better! Communication Cards for Kids & Adults

Kicking Butts: Quit Smoking and Take Charge of Your Health, Second Edition

Lymphedema: Understanding and Managing Lymphedema After Cancer Treatment

What to Eat During Cancer Treatment

When the Focus Is on Care: Palliative Care and Cancer

Emotional Support

Angels & Monsters: A child's eye view of cancer

Cancer in the Family: Helping Children Cope with a Parent's Illness

Chemo and Me: My Hair Loss Experience

Couples Confronting Cancer: Keeping Your Relationship Strong

Crossing Divides: A Couple's Story of Cancer, Hope, and Hiking Montana's Continental Divide

I Can Survive

The Survivorship Net: A Parable for the Family, Friends, and Caregivers of People with Cancer

What Helped Get Me Through: Cancer Survivors Share Wisdom and Hope

Just for Kids

Because . . . Someone I Love Has Cancer: Kids' Activity Book

Healthy Me: A Read-Along Coloring & Activity Book

Imagine What's Possible: Use the Power of Your Mind to Take Control of Your Life During Cancer

Jacob Has Cancer: His Friends Want to Help

Kids' First Cookbook: Delicious-Nutritious Treats To Make Yourself!

Let My Colors Out

The Long and the Short of It: A Tale about Hair

Mom and the Polka-Dot Boo-Boo

Nana, What's Cancer?

No Thanks, but I'd Love to Dance

Our Dad Is Getting Better

Our Mom Has Cancer (hardcover)

Our Mom Has Cancer (paperback)

Our Mom Is Getting Better

What's Up with Bridget's Mom? Medikidz Explain Breast Cancer

What's Up with Jo? Medikidz Explain Brain Tumors

What's Up with Richard? Medikidz Explain Leukemia

What's Up with Lyndon? Medikidz Explain Osteosarcoma

What's Up with Tiffany's Dad? Medikidz Explain Melanoma

Prevention

The American Cancer Society's Healthy Eating Cookbook: A celebration of food, friendship, and healthy living, Third Edition

Celebrate! Healthy Entertaining for Any Occasion

The Great American Eat-Right Cookbook: 140 Great-Tasting, Good-for-You Recipes

Healthy Air: A Read-Along Coloring & Activity Book (25 per pack: Tobacco avoidance)

Healthy Bodies: A Read-Along Coloring & Activity Book (25 per pack: Physical activity)

Healthy Food: A Read-Along Coloring & Activity Book (25 per pack: Nutrition)

National Health Education Standards: Achieving Excellence, Second Edition (available in paperback and on CD-ROM)

Reduce Your Cancer Risk

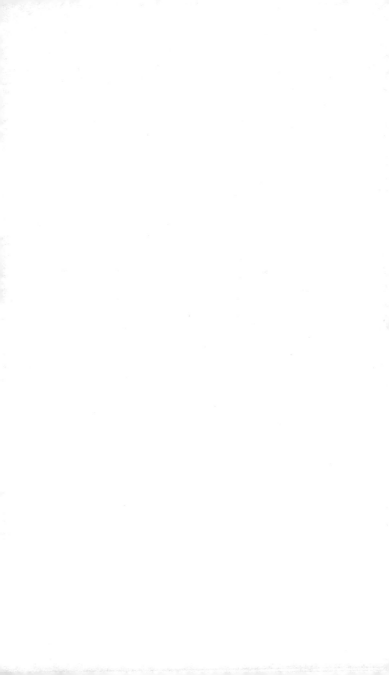

Basal cell carcinoma

Basal cell carcinomas often appear as flat, firm, pale areas, or they may appear as raised pink or red, translucent, shiny, waxy areas. The lesions are prone to bleeding and may contain one or more visible abnormal blood vessels and/or blue, brown, or black areas. Large basal cell carcinomas may have oozing or crusted areas. They can occur anywhere on the body, but usually develop on areas exposed to the sun, especially the head and neck.

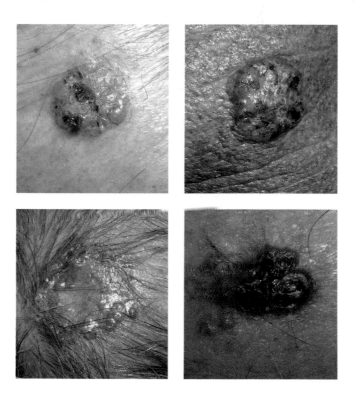

Squamous cell carcinoma

Squamous cell carcinomas may appear as growing lumps, often with a rough, scaly, or crusted surface. They may also appear as flat, reddish patches on the skin that grow slowly. They commonly occur on sun-exposed areas of the body such as the face, ears, neck, lips, and back of the hands. Less frequently, they form on the skin of the genital area. They can also develop on scars or skin ulcers elsewhere on the body.

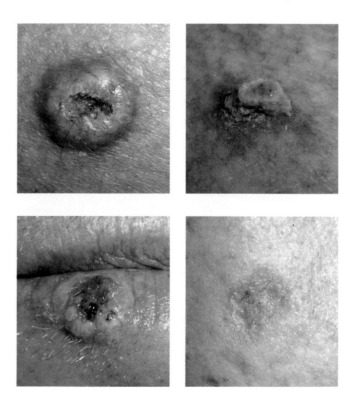

Keratoacanthomas

Keratoacanthomas are fairly common growths that are found on sun-exposed skin. These tumors closely resemble squamous cell carcinomas, and many doctors consider them to be a type of squamous cell cancer. They typically appear as firm, round, flesh-colored or red papules that progress to smooth, shiny dome-shaped nodules. Although they may start as fast-growing lesions, the growth usually slows down. Many keratoacanthomas shrink or even go away on their own over time, without any treatment. However, some continue to grow and a few may even spread to other parts of the body. Their growth is often hard to predict.

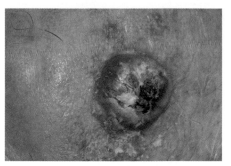

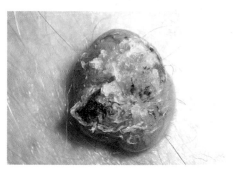

Merkel cell carcinoma

Merkel cell tumors are usually firm pink, red, or purple nodules or ulcers. They are most often found on the head, neck, and arms but can start anywhere. These cancers are believed to be caused in part by sun exposure and partly by Merkel cell polyomavirus (MCV), a common virus that usually causes no symptoms. In a small percentage of people with this infection, changes in the virus's DNA can lead to this form of cancer.

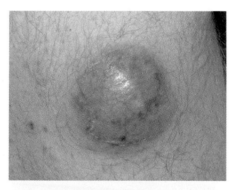

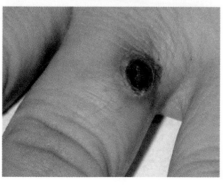

Photos © Paul Nghiem, MD, PhD, and www.merkelcell.org

Actinic keratosis

Actinic keratosis, also known as solar keratosis, is a precancerous skin condition caused by overexposure to the sun. Actinic keratoses are usually small (less than ¼ inch across), rough pinkish-red or flesh-colored spots. They are most common in middle-aged or older adults with fair skin and usually develop on the face, ears, back of the hands, and arms, although they can develop on other parts of the body that have been exposed to the sun. A person with one actinic keratosis usually develops many more.

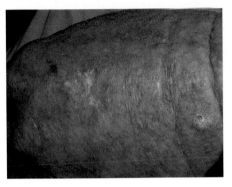

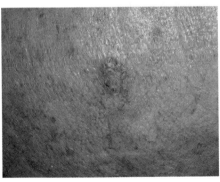

Squamous cell carcinoma in situ (Bowen disease)

Squamous cell carcinoma in situ, also called Bowen disease, is the earliest form of squamous cell skin cancer. "In situ" means that the cells of these cancers are still entirely within the epidermis and have not invaded the dermis. Bowen disease appears as reddish patches. Compared with actinic keratoses, Bowen disease patches tend to be larger (sometimes more than ½ inch across), red, scaly, and sometimes crusted.

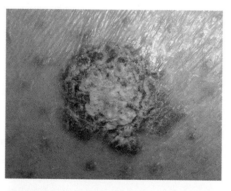

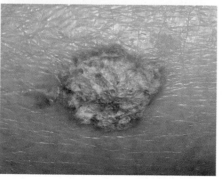

Warts

Warts are rough-surfaced growths caused by a virus called the human papillomavirus (HPV). They are usually harmless, but they can be embarrassing, disfiguring, and may occasionally itch or hurt.

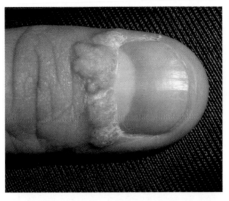

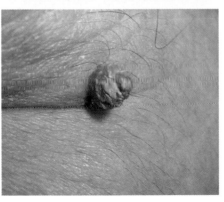

Seborrheic keratosis

Seborrheic keratosis is a benign (noncancerous) wart-like growth on the skin. These lesions often appear as tan, brown, or black raised spots, with a waxy texture or rough surface. They are usually painless but may become irritated and itch. They are often located on the face, chest, shoulders, and back.

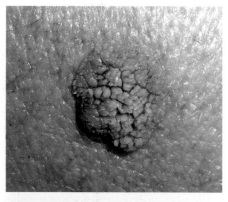

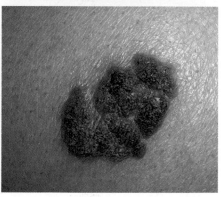